Dictionary of Pharmacy

E. Edwin Jarald
M Pharm, IDCRCT, SMP (PhD)

BR Nahata College of Pharmacy (SIRO) and
BRNSS Contract Research Center
Mandsaur 458001, MP

Sheeja Edwin Jarald
M Pharm, IDCRCT (PhD)

BR Nahata College of Pharmacy (SIRO) and
BRNSS Contract Research Center
Mandsaur 458001, MP

CBSPD

CBS Publishers & Distributors Pvt Ltd

New Delhi • Bengaluru • Chennai • Kochi • Kolkata • Lucknow • Mumbai
Hyderabad • Jharkhand • Nagpur • Patna • Pune • Uttarakhand

Dictionary of Pharmacy

First Edition: 2010
Reprint: 2014, 2016, 2018, 2020, 2023, **2024**

ISBN: 978-81-239-1808-2

Published by Satish Kumar Jain and produced by Varun Jain for

CBS Publishers & Distributors Pvt Ltd

4819/XI Prahlad Street, 24 Ansari Road, Daryaganj, New Delhi 110 002, India.
Ph: 011-23289259, 23266861   Website: www.cbspd.com
                                 e-mail: delhi@cbspd.com

Corporate Office: 204 FIE, Industrial Area, Patparganj, Delhi 110 092
Ph: 011-4934 4934   Fax: 011-4934 4935

                                 e-mail: publishing@cbspd.com; publicity@cbspd.com

Branches

- **Bengaluru:** Seema House 2975, 17th Cross, KR Road, Banasankari 2nd Stage, Bengaluru 560 070, Karnataka, India
  Ph: +91-80-26771678/79   Fax: +91-80-26771680   e-mail: bangalore@cbspd.com
- **Chennai:** 7, Subbaraya Street, Shenoy Nagar, Chennai 600 030, Tamil Nadu, India
  Ph: +91-44-26680620, 26681266   Fax: +91-44-42032115   e-mail: chennai@cbspd.com
- **Kochi:** 42/1325, 1326, Power House Road, Opp KSEB, Power House, Ernakulum Kochi 682 018, Kerala, India
  Ph: +91-484-4059061-65,67   Fax: +91-484-4059065   e-mail: kochi@cbspd.com
- **Kolkata:** 147, Hind Ceramics Compound, 1st Floor, Nilgunj Road, Belghoria, Kolkata-700056, West Bengal, India
  Ph: +033-25633055, 033-25633056   e-mail: kolkata@cbspd.com
- **Lucknow:** Basement, Khushnuma Complex, 7 Meerabai Marg (Behind Jawahar Bhawan), Lucknow-226001, UP, India
  Ph: +0522-4000032   e-mail: tiwari.lucknow@cbspd.com
- **Mumbai:** PWD Shed, Gala no 25/26, Ramchandra Bhatt Marg, Next to JJ Hospital Gate no. 2, Opp. Union Bank of India, Noorbaug, Mumbai-400009, Maharashtra, India
  Ph: 022-66661880/89   e-mail: mumbai@cbspd.com

Representatives

Hyderabad	0-9885175004	Jharkhand	0-9811541605	Nagpur	0-8692091830
Patna	0-9334159340	Pune	0-9664372571	Uttarakhand	0-9716462459

Printed at Sanjay Printers, Sahibabad, U.P, India

Dictionary of

Pharmacy

E. Edwin Jarald
M Pharm, IDCRCT, SMP (PhD)

BR Nahata College of Pharmacy (SIRO) and
BRNSS Contract Research Center
Mandsaur 458001, MP

Sheeja Edwin Jarald
M Pharm, IDCRCT (PhD)

BR Nahata College of Pharmacy (SIRO) and
BRNSS Contract Research Center
Mandsaur 458001, MP

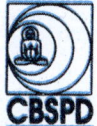

CBS Publishers & Distributors Pvt Ltd

New Delhi • Bengaluru • Chennai • Kochi • Kolkata • Lucknow • Mumbai
Hyderabad • Jharkhand • Nagpur • Patna • Pune • Uttarakhand

We are thankful to God
for giving us the knowledge and power
to come up with such a
dictionary

Preface

Pharmacy is the main cast of modern medicine today, so it is mandatory to know the appropriate meaning of the various terms used along with it. The present book is of great interest as it has a detailed collection of all the technical words which are commonly used in various subjects of pharmacy and applied sciences. The book contains description of more than 4500 words including the terms related to pharmaceutics, chemistry, herbal medicines, biology, plant tissue culture, enzymes and a lot, from simple terms to complex terms. The terms that are commonly found in medical dictionaries are avoided.

There are many dictionaries that already exist in market but we have made an earnest approach in collecting and translating all the terminologies used in different branches of pharmacy so that all the students, researchers, teachers or any one related to pharmaceutical field should be in a position to easily understand the terminology and shall spread his/her knowledge in the right direction with right translation.

Undoubtedly it is a solution for both degree and diploma students of various universities in referring to a range of words related to the respective subject that would provide easy and basic background of information during their course.

We hope all the students and all fellowmen in our field would be benefited through this attempt made by us. We invite your suggestions on this book so that we could make the necessary changes in the forthcoming editions.

E. Edwin Jarald
Sheeja Edwin Jarald

Contents

Dictionary of Pharmacy

A (prefix) Without.

Ab (prefix) Away from.

AB toxins The structure and activity of many exotoxins are based on the AB model. The 'B' portion of the toxin is responsible for toxin binding to a cell and does not directly harm it while the 'A' portion enters the cell and disrupts its function.

Abaxial Surface of any structure which is remote or turned away from the axis, such as the lower surface of a leaf.

Abbreviated new drug application (ANDA) It was established under the Drug Price Competition and Patent Term Restoration Act (1984) and allowed the FDA to accept abbreviated new drug applications for generic versions of drugs first approved after 1962. If the drug was generically equivalent to brand name drugs already proven to be safe and effective, safety and effectiveness data are not required to be submitted.

Abciss Detach, separate from main structure.

Abdomen The posterior body division of an arthropod.

Abduction A sketching away of an arm or leg from the middle line of the body.

Aberration Deviation from that which is normal or an imperfection on an optical lens resulting in a disturbed image.

Abietic acid Organic acid prepared by isomerization of rosin, which is used in the manufacture of soaps, lacquers and lastics.

Abiogenesis The spontaneous generation of biological cells not including known biological explanation or early theory that held that some organisms originated from nonliving material.

Abiotic disease A disease caused by factors other than pathogens.

Abirritant An agent used to reduce irritation.

Ablution Washing.

Abnormal hemoglobin Hemoglobin molecule with a different shape due to an altered amino acid sequence that is caused by an altered DNA base sequence, e.g. sickle-cell anemia.

ABO antigens Innate blood group compounds significant for blood typing and transfusions.

Abortifacient Agent that induces abortion, miscarriage, or premature expulsion of a fetus.

Abortive Same as abortifacient.

Abradant Agent that abrades or scrapes.

Abrasion Scraping of the mucous membranes, teeth or skin.

Abrasive Material used to scrape or erode a surface.

Abscess Accumulation of pus in any part of the body.

Abscisic acid Growth inhibiting plant hormone (a sesquiterpene) which is present in a variety of plant organs such as leaves buds, fruits, seeds and tubers. Promotes senescence and abscission of leaves, induced dormancy in buds and seed. Antagonizes influence of growth promoting hormones. This harmone acts by inhibiting nucleic acid and protein synthesis.

Abscissa Horizontal axis of a graph or plot.

Abscission The normal shedding from a plant of an organ that is mature or aged, e.g. a ripe fruit, an old leaf.

Absolute bioavailability Absolute bioavailability (F) is the fraction of drug systemically absorbed from the dosage form F is calculated as the ratio of the AUC for the dosage form given orally to the AUC obtained after intravenous (IV) drug administration (adjusted for dose).

Absolute configuration The spatial display of the atoms of a chiral molecular entity or group and their stereochemical description.

Absolute temperature An expression of fundamental heat intensity, $°T = °C + 273.15$, its synonym is degrees Kelvin.

Absolute time Refers to one of the two types of geologic time (relative time being the other), with a definite age date established mostly by the decay of radioactive elements, although ages may also be obtained by counting tree rings, decay of a specific type of atom, or annual sedimentary layers (such as varves in lakes or layers in a glacier).

Absolute unit Measurable dimension that is defined by internationally agreed-upon standards, e.g. kilogram, second, meter.

Absolute zero A hypothetical temperature characterized by a complete absence of heat and

approximately equivalent to– 59.67°F or –273.15°C.

Absolutes Values or dimensions that are defined by international agreement.

Absorb To take in food and drugs from the intestinal tract, or to take in and become a fraction of an existing whole.

Absorbance Capacity of a layer of a substance to absorb radiation.

Absorbent Any substance that promotes absorption, soaks up liquid, or acts as a sponge.

Absorption band An area in an absorption spectrum of a material in which the absorptivity reaches the upper limit.

Absorption bases Absorption bases are anhydrous and water-insoluble. Therefore, they are not washable in water, although they can absorb water.

Absorption cell Vessel used to hold substances for determination of their absorption spectra, e.g. cuvette in spectrophotometry.

Absorption coefficient A measure of the rate of decrease in the intensity of electromagnetic radiation after it passes through a particular material or absorption of one substance into another.

Absorption ointment base An ointment base which is able to absorb and hold relatively large amounts of water (e.g. lanolin).

Absorption, active Movement of any substances through a living membrane in opposition to a concentration gradient, e.g. an energy requiring process catalyzed by enzymes.

Absorption, facilitated Movement of any substances through membranes supported by a carrier.

Absorption, passive Movement of any substances through membranes by simple diffusion.

Absorption It is a biological process by which drugs and other substances are transported across body membranes.

Absorptive feeders Animals such as tapeworms that ingest food through the body wall.

Abstinence Drug or any other substance been denied by the person himself.

Abstraction Removal of one or more ingredients from a mixture or a mental state illustrated by a total isolation from its environment.

Acacia gum It is a dried gummy exudate of the acacia tree, used as an emulsifying or suspending agent.

Acalymmate Refers to pollen tetrad or polyad, when the ectexine is separately differentiated on each grain, there being no common covering of the pollen mass.

Acaulescent Having no stem or seemingly without a stem.

Acceleration of gravity Attractive force of gravity which results in the rate of increase in movement of a substance 980.665 cm/sec^2.

Acceleration Rate of increase in the velocity of movement of any particle or an object, usually expressed in cm/sec^2.

Acceptance sampling The statistically supported quality control methods of picking a representative part of a lot of pharmaceutical preparations.

Accessory bud(s) One or more buds other than the normal single bud occurring in the leaf axil.

Accessory cell Subsidiary cell.

Accessory flower parts Sepals and petals found on flowers. The sepals and petals are not essential for pollination but may aid in attracting insects or other organisms.

Accessory fruits Fruits, whether derived from a single flower or several, with tissue that is other than carpellary in origin.

Acclimatization The biological process in which an organism becomes accustomed to a new environment.

Accommodation schedule A schedule that defines all areas that can influence unit operations required for manufacturing, and relationships and flows between them.

Accrescent Continuing to increase in size after maturity, as the calyx of some plants after flowering.

Accrete Practice of adding up a new enrollees to a health plan.

Accumbent Embryo that is folded so that the radicle lies against the edges of the two cotyledons.

Acetaldehyde CH_3CHO an intermediate in the aerobic and anaerobic respiration of carbohydrates. Retards or inhibits germination and growth of some fungi.

Acetate A salt, ester or the conjugate base of acetic acid.

Acetogenins Polyketides derived from acetate with 35:37 carbon atoms in a single almost unbranched chain, substituted by 6:8 oxygen atoms.

Acetyl CoA (acetyl coenzyme A). A compound having acetyl combined through a sulphur bridge with coenzyme A. The formation of acetyl CoA is an energy-consuming reaction which involves the conservation of ATP to AMP and pyrophosphate. It is a degradation product of fatty acids, carbohydrates and some amino acids.

Acetylcholine It is a neurotransmitter released at neuromuscular junctions. It has empirical formula $C_7H_{17}NO_3$. It transmits a signal to an adjacent nerve or muscle cell by binding to receptors on the target cell surface.

Acetylcholinesterase (AChE) An enzyme present in various tissues, including muscle and red cells, that breaks down acetylcholine (a chemical released by nerves that activates muscle contractions) and helps to maintain proper transmission of impulses between nerve cells and between nerve cells and muscles.

Acetylenes The simplest of a class of triple-bonded hydrocarbons.

Acetyl-S-CoA An intermediate, which is produced by coenzyme A when it gets detached carbon dioxide from the a-keto-acid during respiration.

Achene Means a simple, one-seeded fruit in which the seed is attached to the ovary wall at only one point, such as the "seed" on the surface of a strawberry.

Achlamydeous Related to flower, lacking a perianth parts, usually best to describe as such.

Acicular (In Latin, acicula means a small needle) slender and

pointed; needle-like and with a sharp point.

Acid A compound of an electronegative radical or element with hydrogen; it forms salts by substituting a part or all of the hydrogen with an electropositive radical or element (compound that gives off H^+ ions in solution).

Acid-base balance Relative concentrations of acids and bases as in an organism or a physical system.

Acid-base indicator A dye solution that alters its color with changes in pH.

Acidity constant Ionization constant of a weak acid.

Acid dyes Dyes that are anionic or have negatively charged groups like carboxyls.

Acid-fast A staining property shown by some of the bacteria that are not decolorized by mineral acids after staining with aniline dyes.

Acid feed To adjust the pH or an injection of an acid into a liquid stream to make it less alkaline.

Acid ionization constant The degree to which an acid ionizes.

Acid phosphatase An enzyme found primarily in the prostate and semen. Increased blood serum levels may indicate cancer of the prostate or may follow prostatic massage.

Acid rain The precipitation of sulfuric acid and other acids as rain. The acids form when sulfur dioxide and nitrogen oxides released during the combustion of fossil fuels combine with water and oxygen in the atmosphere.

Acid value Number of milligrams of potassium hydroxide required to neutralize the free fatty acids present in one gram of substance.

Acid, weak An organic acid that does not totally dissociate in water.

Acidity function Any function that measures the thermodynamic hydron-accepting or donating capacity of a solvent system.

Acidifier An herb or substance that increases or imparts acidity, or lessens alkalinity, to the body fluids, especially the blood or the urine.

Acidimetry Quantitative estimation of total amount of acid in a sample by titrating it with standard base.

Acidophile A microorganism that has its optimum growth at pH between 0 and 5.5.

Acidosis An unusually increased concentration of acid in an organism; lowering of the pH of the blood below the normal of 7.4 due to an increase in acid metabolites.

Acne Chronic inflammatory condition of the sebaceous glands mainly involving the face, back and chest.

Acneiform Lesion that resembles acne.

Acoelomates Animals that do not have a coelom or body cavity, e.g. sponges and flatworms.

Acoustic It pertains to hearing.

Acquired immune deficiency syndrome (AIDS) An infectious disease/syndrome caused by the human immunodeficiency virus and is characterized by the loss of a normal immune response, followed by increased susceptibility to opportunistic infections and an increased risk of some cancers.

Acquired immunity A type of specific immunity that develops after exposure to a specific antigen or if the antibodies are transferred from one individual to another.

Acrid An herb or substance that has a hot biting taste, or causes heat and irritation when applied to the skin.

Acrodromous Palmate leaf venation, with two or more primary or strongly developed secondary veins running in convergent arches towards the apex.

Acromegaly Chronic disease that is characterized by enlarged face and hands due to the hypersecretion of the pituitary growth hormone.

Acropetal Developing upward from the base toward the apex.

ACTH Adrenocorticotropic hormone; a hormone secreted by the pituitary gland to stimulate the adrenal glands to produce glucocorticoid hormones.

Actin The protein from which microfilaments are composed, forms the contractile filaments of sarcomeres in muscle cells.

Actinobacteria A group of gram-positive bacteria containing the actinomycetes and their high G 1 C relatives.

Actinocytic Stomata, with five or more somewhat radially enlarged or elongated subsidiary cells surrounding the guard cells.

Actinodromous Palmate leaf venation, with three or more primary veins arising from at or near the base, ascending or diverging, whether or not reaching the margin.

Actinomorphic Descriptive of a flower or set of flower parts which can be cut through the center into equal and similar parts along two or more planes; having radial symmetry.

Actinomycete It is an aerobic, gram-positive bacterium that forms hyphae and asexual spores.

Actinomycosis Fatal, chronic, fungal disease with multiple abscesses that form draining sinuses and lesions on neck, face, lungs and abdomen.

Actinostele It is an alternative of a protostele in which the xylem forms a more or less star-shaped central mass, with phloem between the arms.

Action point A value set to make out when a parameter has glided outside the acceptance criteria.

Action potential A reversal of the electrical potential in the plasma membrane of a neuron that occurs when a nerve cell is stimulated. This is caused by rapid changes in membrane permeability to sodium and potassium.

Activated carbon It is formed from wood, pulp-mill char, etc. and is used to adsorb organic impurities from water.

Activated charcoal Carbon black that has been treated with superheated steam to expel the adsorbed gases so that the adsorptive powers increases.

Activated support A support matrix capable of covalently binding a molecule.

Activation energy Energy needed to initiate a chemical reaction.

Active center The location where the specific reaction takes place in an enzyme.

Active carrier An individual who has an evident clinical case of a disease and can transmit the infection to others.

Active immunity The formation of antibody that can be stimulated by vaccination or infection.

Active immunization The generation of active immunity by natural exposure to a pathogen or by vaccination.

Active ingredient Any component that is intended to provide pharmacological activity or effect directly in the mitigation, cure, treatment, diagnosis, or prevention of disease, or have influence on the structure or function of the human or in animal body.

Active ingredient/constituent (herbs) One or more molecules which have been isolated from the plants and scientifically established to have a specific physiological activity, both in isolation and within the context of the whole herb or extract. They generally exhibit a dose dependent response.

Active site The region of a protein molecule that binds the specific substrate and modifies it chemically to form a new product in an enzyme or interacts with it in a receptor.

Active transport Energy-requiring transport of a solution across a membrane towards increasing concentration.

Active tubular secretion It means the active transport of the acidic molecules from the blood into the lumen of the renal.

Actual yield It is the quantity that has actually been produced at any suitable phase of processing, manufacture or packaging of a drug product.

Acumen The point of an acuminate leaf.

Acuminate Drawn out into a long point, tapering point.

Acupressure The principle of acupuncture has been used by the ancient Chinese; technique involves the use of finger pressure on specific points along the body to treat diseases like aches, pains, arthritis, stress, etc.

Acupuncture A healthy energy balance is restored by inserting fine needle at specific points to stimulate, disperse and regulate the flow of vital energy.

Acupuncture points Refer to the anatomic points on the body used in acupuncture.

Acute A condition that occurs suddenly for a short period of time.

Acute (leaf apex) Ending in a sharp point.

Acyl-CoA A product of fatty acid activation. Acyl-CoA is subsequently carried by carnitine into the mitochondria for beta-oxidation.

Acyl-CoA synthetase An enzyme that converts a fatty acid to acyl-CoA for subsequent beta oxidation.

Adaptation Adjustment of an organism by an environment so that it becomes better fitted for a particular environment.

Adaptive radiation The development of a variety of species from a single ancestral form; occurs when a new habitat becomes available to a population.

Adaptogen A substance that invigorates or strengthens the system. Also known as tonic.

Adaxial Situated toward the axis, frequently on the upper side of branch.

Addition reaction A chemical reaction of two or more reacting molecular entities, resulting in a single reaction product containing all atoms of all components, with formation of two chemical bonds and a net reduction in bond multiplicity in at least one of the reactants. The reverse process is called an elimination reaction.

Additional drug benefit list A list of pharmaceutical products approved by a health plan and employer for dispensing in larger quantities than the standards covered under a benefit package in order to facilitate long-term patient use.

Adduction The movement of a limb or eye toward the median plane of the body.

Adenine (A) 6-aminopurine (purine base), occurring in DNA and RNA and also a component of adenosine triphosphate.

Adenosine diphosphate It is the diphosphate ester of adenosine. It is related to adenosine triphosphate in the transfer of energy through 'high energy' bonds during the respiration of carbohydrates. The energy gets released in the production of ester phosphates by the ADP that acts as a phosphorylating agent.

Adenosine monophosphate A phosphorylated nucleoside having the purine, adenine and the sugar ribose phosphorylated in 5 position. It acts in the regulation of glucolysis and gluconeogenesis, thereby promoting the formation of fructose biphosphate from fructose-6-phosphate (i.e. promoting glycolysis) at the same time inhibits the back reaction to fructose biphosphate.

Adenosine triphosphate (ATP) A common form in which energy is stored in living systems; consists of a nucleotide (with ribose sugar) with three phosphate groups.

Adherent Closely attached.

Adhesion Attachment or sticking or holding of tissue to one another.

Adhesive tape Strip of material that sticks or adheres to skin.

Adipose tissue Tissue that contains fats and fat cells.

Adiposis Refers to the accumulation of excess fat in the body.

Adjunct Additional substances added to the drug to make a finished drug dosage form. Example, lactose as a filler for capsules.

Adjuvant Excipients added to a drug formulation to improve the manufacturing process, product quality, or pharmacological action, e.g. carboxymethylcellulose to aid in suspending drug particles in a liquid.

ADME Abbreviation for absorption, distribution, metabolism, excretion.

Admedial Towards the midline of the lamina.

Adnate Fusion of different structures or parts.

Adrenaline A neurohormone secreted by the adrenal medulla and is a potent endogenous stimulant.

Adrenergic Pertains to the sympathetic nervous system.

Adrenergic agent Means a chemical compound that exerts its principal pharmacological effect by stimulation of peripheral sites

of the sympathetic part of the autonomic nervous system.

Adrenergic blocking agent A drug that blocks impulses at the sympathetic receptor.

Adrenocortex hormones These are steroids secreted from adrenal cortex, which might have either male or female sex hormone activity or glucocorticoid or mineralocorticoid.

Adrenocorticotrophic hormone Peptide hormone that is secreted by the anterior lobe of the pituitary gland that stimulates the adrenal cortex to secrete adrenocorticosteroids

Adson syndrome Means compression of the brachial plexus leading to sensory disturbance of the upper extremity, also known as "Naffziger syndrome".

Adsorbate Substance that is adsorbed on a surface of an adsorbent.

Adsorbent Any material that adsorbs other substances.

Adsorption Adhesion of the molecules of a gas, liquid or dissolved substance to a surface because of chemical or electrical attraction—typically accomplished with granular activated carbon to remove dissolved organics and chlorine. Also refers to the attachment of charged particles to the chemically active groups on the surface and in the pores of an ion exchanger.

Adulterant An impure ingredient or a substitute product added into a preparation.

Adventitious Irregular and secondarily produced, it is not a primary part.

Adventitious roots A root, which grows from somewhere other than the primary root, e.g. roots that arise from stems or leaves.

Adventive Refers to the plants that are not native to the environment.

Adverse effects Toxic effects due to the exposure to a drug or medical device.

Adverse drug reaction (ADR) An undesired effect that may be caused by a drug.

Aerenchyma Parenchyma tissue with large and abundant intercellular air spaces (air storing tissue). It resembles the tissue of cork.

Aerial root Arising above ground, often from an axil that means for the plant to absorb moisture from the air.

Aerobe An organism that can live and grow only in the presence of oxygen.

Aerobia Plural of aerobe.

Aerobic Living in air.

Aerobic anoxygenic photosynthesis This is a photosynthetic process in which electron donors do not result in oxygen evolution like organic matter or sulfide.

Aerobic bacteria Refers to bacteria capable of growing in the presence of oxygen.

Aerobic respiration It is a metabolic process in which molecules, frequently organic, are oxidized with oxygen as the final electron acceptor.

Aerosol A product that is dispensed by a propellant from a metal can up to a maximum size of 33.8 fluid ounces (1000 ml) or a glass or plastic bottle up to a size of 4 fluid ounces (118.3 ml). They are designed to deliver drug systemically or topically with the aid of a liquefied or propelled gas.

Aerosol photometer Light-scattering mass concentration representing instrument with a threshold sensitivity of at least 10 to the negative third power micro-gram per liter for 0.3 µm diameter DOP (dioctyl phthalate) concentrations over a range of 10 to the fifth power times the threshold sensitivity. These photometers may include hand-held remote meter probes that can scan for air-borne contaminants in HEPA filters, in penetrations around frames, seals and plenums, and in hoods and work stations.

Aestivation The arrangement of sepals and petals or their lobes relative to one another in an unexpanded flower bud.

Aetheroleum Refers to the essential or volatile oil as a distinct aromatic product obtained from the plant.

Affinity It is the tendency of a molecule to associate with another.

Aflatoxin A polyketide secondary fungal metabolite from Aspergillus species that can cause cancer.

Agamospermy It is a kind of apomictic reproduction, the enlargement of seeds from ovules without fertilization.

Aga A complex mixture of polysaccharides obtained from marine red algae, used as an emulsion stabilizer in foods, as a sizing in cloths, as a gelling agent and as a solid substrate or media for the laboratory culture of microorganisms. Agar melts at 100°C and when cooled below 44°C forms a stiff and transparent gel. Microbes are seeded and grown on the surface of the gel.

Agarose Refers to a highly purified form of agar.

Agarose gel electrophoresis This
is a method used to separate,
identify, and purify molecules of
different molecular weight and/or
structure. It is specially applied to
the separation of protein or DNA
fragments where it is rapid,
simple, and accurate, and these
separated molecules can be
visualized directly after staining
with dyes. The migration rate of
molecules through agarose gel is
dependent on the following
parameters like molecular size,
agarose concentration, molecular
conformation and electric current.

Agene Refers to nitrogen trichloride (NCl_3).

Agglomerate Agglomerates are
suspended solids gathered together to form larger clumps or
masses that are easier to remove
by filtration or settling.

Agglutination The sticking together of insoluble antigens such
as bacteria, viruses or erythrocytes by a particular antibody.
Agglutination assays are used to
decide the type of human blood
before a transfusion.

Aggregate Crowded into a cluster.

Aggregate fruit A cluster of fruits
formed from the free carpels of
one flower. Also known as compound fruit.

Aglycone The non-carbohydrate
group of a glycoside that comes
out on its hydrolysis (at times
called aglucone).

Agonist An agonist is a substance
or a drug that can interact with
a receptor and initiate a physiological or a pharmacological response characteristic of that
receptor.

Agrobacterium A type of soil-
inhabiting bacteria that is
capable of introducing DNA from
plasmids in the bacteria into the
genome of plant cells which is
frequently used in genetic
transformation of plants.

Ague Type of fever marked by
chills and shivering.

AHF (antihemophilic factor)
Comes under the clotting of blood
and it is also known as factor VIII.

**Air-borne particulate cleanliness
classes** Statistically allowable
number of particles equal to, or
larger than 0.5μm in size per
cubic foot of air.

Air cleaners Filtration systems
that may be unattached or
installed in a ceiling or wall to
remove contaminants such as
bacteria, viruses, and dust from
the air. Air cleaners may include
HEPA filters.

Air flow visualization Method of
using chemical smoke or fog to
visualize flow patterns in a clean
room or clean space.

Air-lift bioreactor A reactor in
which the source of agitation is
air sparged upwards through a
draft tube. This is most widely
used for cell culture applications
and monoclonal antibody production.

Airlock A room or space considered to act as a means of
separating areas of different air
classification or quality. It may
contain a technique to remove
particulate contamination from
clean room garments as personnel pass through, and usually
incorporates HEPA filtered air
supply and interlocking doors.

Air suspension-coated tablets
Air suspension-coated tablets are

fed into a vertical cylinder and supported by a column of air that enters from the bottom of the cylinder. As the coating solution enters the system, it is rapidly applied to the suspended, rotating solids.

Air velocity meters/monitors Meters used to measure and indicate the force and speed of air flow.

Akaryotic Without a true nucleus.

Akinete Enlarged cell with food reserves and thick cell wall which may undergo dormancy.

Alanine It is a non-polar amino acid.

Albinism It is a genetic condition caused by the body's inability to produce pigments; an autosomal recessive trait.

Albino A pigmentless white phenotype which is determined by a mutation in a gene coding for a pigment-synthesizing enzyme.

Albumen Endosperm.

Albumin The white of egg is a simple protein widely distributed throughout the tissues and fluid of plants and animals, known as albumin. It is soluble in pure water. It precipitates from a solution by mineral acids, and coagulable by heat in acid or neutral solution.

Albuminoid Resembles albumin, a simple protein that is present in horny and cartilaginous tissues. It is insoluble in neutral solvents. Few examples are keratin, elastin and collagen.

Alcohol sulphuris It Means carbon disulfide.

Alcoholic fermentation An anaerobic step that yeast use after glycolysis that breaks down pyruvic acid to ethanol and carbon dioxide.

Aldehyde dehydrogenase They are enzymes which oxidize a wide variety of aliphatic and aromatic aldehydes using NADP as a cofactor.

Aldehydes Aldehydes have a general formula of R – CHO and contain a carbonl group (C = O).

Aldose It is a monosaccharide sugar that has an aldehyde (CHO) group in the first position and a CHOH group of the second position.

Aldosterone It is a hormone secreted by the adrenal glands that controls the reabsorption of sodium in the renal tubule of the nephron.

Alembroth, salt of A double chloride of mercury and ammonium

Aleurone Proteins in living cells.

Algae A division of the Thallophyta, which includes the holophytic members. All are aquatic, or sub-aquatic, and vary from the unicellular types to the large sea weeds. They lack any vascular tissue, and are not differentiated into stem, root and leaf. The reproductive organs are essentially one-celled, and the gametes are mostly flagellate.

Algaroth Antimony oxychloride, SbOCl. It is an emetic.

Algin The magnesium-calcium salt of alginic acid which occurs in inner cell-wall of the brown algae. Commercially, it is used in the manufacture of confectionary and to some extent in the manufacture of fibres.

Alginate Refers to salt form of alginic acid, a polysaccharide colloid produced in walls of

Phaeophyceae made of mannuronic acid and glucuronic acid units.

Alginic acid It is a carbohydrate polymer which is made up of D-mannuronic acid and L-glucuronic acid units. Found mainly in cell walls of brown algae where it functions as agent of ion exchange.

Alien species A species, subspecies, or lower taxon introduced outside its original distribution area. In plants, it incorporates any part, gametes, seeds, eggs, or propagules of such species that might survive and consequently reproduce.

Aliform Refers to paratracheal axial parenchyma, the parenchyma cells associated with the vessels forming a wing-shaped mass in transverse section.

Aliquot Pertaining to an exact divisor or factor of a quantity, specially of a figure. To separate out a sample to several containers for several analytical tests.

Alkahest It is a universal solvent.

Alkaline Means basic, having a pH greater than 7.

Alkalinity An expression of the total amount of basic anions (hydroxyl groups) in a solution.

Alkaloids They are organic, nitrogenous containing bases, usually with a heterocyclic ring of some kind. The three main categories are: 1. true alkaloids: nitrogen containing heterocyclic compounds derived from an amino acid, e.g. tropane alkaloids, quinolizidine alkaloids, 2. protoalkaloids: derived from amino acids, but lacking a heterocyclic ring, 3. pseudoalkaloids: derived

from terpenes, sterols, aliphatic acids, nicotinic acid, or purines.

Alkanes Alkanes, which are also called paraffins or saturated hydrocarbons, have a general formula of $R - CH_2 - CH_3$, where R is a radical or molecule fragment.

Alkannin It is a naphthoquinone derived from the p-hydroxybenzoic acid pathway.

Alkenes Alkenes, also called olefins or unsaturated hydrocarbons, have a general formula of $R - CH = 5CH_2$.

Alkyl halides Alkyl halides, also known as halogenated hydrocarbons, have a general formula of $R - CH_2 - X$.

Alkylating agent A chemical agent that can add alkyl groups, like ethyl or methyl groups to another molecule.

Allantoic fluid The white portion of an egg.

Allele One of a pair or more of alternative hereditary characters; a gene which can occupy the same locus as another gene in a particular chromosome (alternate forms of a gene).

Allelochemicals Compounds that have an allelopathic effect.

Allelocytic Refers to stomata, with an alternating complex of three or more C shaped subsidiary cells of graded sizes surrounding the guard cells.

Allelopathy The ability of a plant species to produce substances that are toxic to certain other plants.

Allergen A substance that aggravates an allergic response.

Allergenic extract An extract of a substance that causes an allergic reaction.

Allergy The body's reaction to any foreign substance to which a person may be sensitive. The reactions can range from mild to severe and life-threatening.

Alligation alternate A method for calculation of the number of parts of two or more components of known concentration to be mixed when the final desired concentration is known.

Alligation medial A method for calculating the average concentration of a mixture of two or substances.

Allitol A carbohydrate product resulting from the reduction of the aldehyde functional group in D-allose.

Allium compounds Also known as organosulfides, or allyl sulfides, found in allium vegetables, which include garlic, onions, leeks, chives and shallots. Allium compounds may boost enzyme cancer detox systems and prevent bacteria from converting nitrates into substances that help make carcinogens.

Allogamy Fertilisation involving gametes from different flowers or plants.

Alloparasite Parasite that is not related to its host.

Allopathy The treatment of disease by creating conditions that are opposite or hostile to the conditions resulting from the disease itself; from Greek roots meaning other and disease. Drugs and surgery are allopathic treatments. The term is sometimes used to refer to conventional Western medicine to contrast it with alternative therapies.

Allopolyploid A plant with a chromosome number that is the pro

duct of the addition of the diploid numbers of the parent plants. It may be due to hybridisation.

Allowable depletion The proportion of available water that can be used before irrigation is needed.

Allozyme It is a form of an enzyme which differs in amino acid sequence, as shown by electrophoretic mobility or some other property, from other forms of the same enzyme and is encoded by one allele at a single locus.

Alluvial soil A soil that is derived from marine, estuarine or river deposits. Generally has a high fertility.

Allyl group It is a functional group composed of $H_2C=CH:CH_2:R$, found in many of the sulfur compounds of Allium species as well as in other organic molecules.

Allylic substitution reaction This is a substitution reaction occurring at position 1/ of an allylic system, the double bond being between positions 2/ and 3/. The arriving group may be attached to the same atom 1/ as the leaving group, or the incoming group becomes attached at the relative position 3/, with movement of the double bond from 2/3 to 1/2.

Alopecia A general term referring to hair loss of any cause.

Alpha carotene It is a powerful antioxidant carotenoid that the body converts to vitamin A, when required.

Alpha decay A type of radioactive decay in which a radioisotope emits a large but slow-moving particle consisting of two protons and two neutrons.

Alpha-linolenic acid It is an omega-3 fatty acid that serves as the parent compound in the synthesis of other omega-3 fatty acids in the body and is also known as essential fatty acid.

Alpha tocopherol It is the most common form of vitamin E, found in the human body and in supplements.

Alterative An herb or substance that corrects body functions either gradually or quickly by stimulating the defensive mechanisms of the metabolism, blood, or tissue in the presence of chronic or acute disease. (The time required may be six months or longer if chronic or a few minutes if acute.).

Alternate Branched at different levels on opposite sides of main axis.

Alternation of generations Life cycle in which haploid and diploid generations interchange with each other.

Alternative medicine Any form of therapy used alone, without suggested standard/conventional treatment.

Altitudinal gradient As altitude increases, a gradient of cooler, drier conditions occurs.

Alum It is aluminum sulfate, commonly added during municipal water treatment to cause insoluble colloids to coalesce into larger particles that can be removed by settling.

Alveola A small pit on the surface of an organ.

Alveolate Pitted form or honeycombed on the surface.

Alveoli Tiny, thin-walled, inflatable sacs in the lungs where oxygen and carbon dioxide are exchanged.

Alzheimer's disease A disease that causes memory loss, perso-nality changes, dementia and, ultimately, death. Genes have been found for familial forms of Alzheimer's disease.

Ambient The normal environment conditions such as temperature, relative humidity, or room pressure of a particular area under consideration.

Ames test A bacterial test for carcinogens.

Amides Amides have a general formula $R - CONH_2$ or $R - CONR - R$ (lactum form).

Amine A substance that may be derived from ammonia by the replacement of one or more of the hydrogen atoms by hydrocarbon radicals. Amines contain an amino group ($-NH_2$). The amino group can exist in ionized or un-ionized form.

Amino acids Any of a group of twenty hydrocarbon molecules (containing the radical group NH_2) linked jointly in various combinations to form proteins in living things. There are 21 'standard' amino acids from which proteins are formed, and many additional modified types.

Amino acid residue (in a polypeptide) When two or more amino acids join to form a peptide, the elements of water are removed, and what remains of each amino acid is called as an amino acid residue.

Amino acid sequence Also known as the primary structure of a protein/polypeptide; the sequence of amino acids in a protein/polypeptide controlled by the sequence of DNA bases.

Amino group A nitrogen atom single-bonded to two hydrogen atoms.

Aminoglycosides A division of antibiotics specific for gram-negative bacteria.

Aminotransferase An enzyme who's increased concentration sometimes result in the elevation of toxic ammonia levels.

Ammonia The common name for NH_3, a strongly basic, irritating, colourless gas which is lighter than air and readily soluble in water.

Ammonium vandate Used for the detection of alkaloids, phenolic compounds and steroids.

Amnesic shellfish poisoning The disease occurring in humans and animals that eat seafood contaminated with domoic acid from diatoms. The disease produces short-term memory loss.

Amniotic fluid The fluid surrounding the developing fetus which is found within the amniotic sac contained in the mother's womb.

Amoeboid movement Moving by means of cytoplasmic flow and the formation of pseudopodia, i.e. temporary cytoplasmic protrusions of the cytoplasm.

Amoebicidal Drug for amoebic dysentery.

Amoebocytes Amoeboid cells in sponges that occur in the matrix between the epidermal and collar cells. They transport nutrients.

Amorphous Lacks definite structure or shape.

Amphibians These are a class of terrestrial vertebrates which lay their eggs and also mate in water but live on land as adults following a juvenile stage where they live in water and breathe through gills.

Amphibious Refers to the general habitat, a plant growing both in water and on land.

Amphicarpy Produces two kinds of fruit, both aerial and subterranean.

Amphicribral Refers to vascular bundles with phloem completely surrounding the xylem.

Amphimixis Reproducing sexually.

Amphiphloic It is a variant of a siphonostele in which there is phloem both outside and inside the xylem.

Amphistomatic Refers to leaves in which stomata are borne on both sides.

Amphitrichous Having a flagellum at each end of the cell.

Amphitropous Refers to ovule which is bending both ways on the stalk.

Amphivasal Vascular bundles, with xylem completely surrounding the phloem.

Ampholyte Electrolyte that can either give up or take on a hydrogen ion and can thus behave as either an acid or a base.

Amphoteric Having two opposite characteristics is known as amphoteric.

Amplexicaul Refers to base of leaf, clasping and more or less encircling the stem yet free from it.

Amplification An increase in the number of copies of a specific DNA fragment, that can be *in vivo* or *in vitro*.

Ampoule or ampule A small glass vial sealed after filling and one of the first devices developed for safe storage of sterile injectable unit.

Amylase An enzyme that is responsible for the breakdown of starch and it is part of the diastase complex. O-amylase attacks the amylase part of the starch molecule first, breaking it down to maltose. α-amylase attacks the remaining part of the molecule, any amylase breaking it down to dextrins (5–10 glucose units), which get further attacked by the β-amylase.

Amylopectin It is a polysaccharide made up of branched chains containing a large number of glucose units linked in 1:4 or 1:6 position.

Amyloplast It is a colorless organelle linked to starch production.

Amylose It is a long straight-chained polysaccharide that is made up of about 300 glucose units linked in the 1:4 position. Also it is a constituent of starch, and is responsible for the typical blue colour of starches when treated with iodine solution.

Amyotrophic lateral sclerosis A hereditary, fatal degenerative nerve disorder, also known as Lou Gehrig's disease.

Ana Refers to the apertures of pollen grains, located at or towards the distal pole.

ANA Abbreviation for antinuclear antibodies. These antibodies react to an individual's own tissue who is suffering from autoimmune disease.

Anabolic Refers to synthesis, opposite of catabolic.

Anabolic reactions Reactions in cells in which new chemical bonds are formed and new molecules are made.

Anabolism The intracellular process implicated in the synthesis of more complex compounds than those involved in catabolism and requires energy.

Anaerobes Microorganisms that thrive best only when deprived of oxygen.

Anaerobic Living without free oxygen, in a reducing atmosphere (organisms that are not dependent on oxygen for respiration).

Anaerobic bacteria Bacteria that are capable of growing in the absence of oxygen.

Anaerobic respiration The enzymatic breakdown of a substrate releasing energy, without using oxygen. The anaerobic respiration of a given weight of a substrate gives out less energy than the aerobic respiration of the same weight of the same substrate.

Analgesic An herb or substance that relieves or reduces pain without causing unconsciousness.

Analog An analog is a drug whose structure is related to that of another drug but whose chemical and biological properties may be quite dissimilar.

Analogous enzymes Refer to structurally unrelated enzymes that catalyse the same reaction.

Analogous structures Body parts, which serve the same function in different organisms, but differ in structure and embryological development, e.g. the wings of insects and birds.

Analysis of variance (ANOVA) A basic statistical technique for analyzing experimental data. It is used to test whether the means of many samples differ but it does so using variation instead of mean.

Analyte A substance that is undergoing analysis or is being measured.

Analytical method Small scale process used to identify, characterize and/or separate a mixture, a compound, or an unknown material into its constituent parts or elements.

Anaphase It is a phase of mitosis in which the chromosomes begin to separate.

Anaphrodisiac A herb or substance that reduces or represses sexual desire or potency.

Anaphylatoxin A substance capable of releasing histamine from mast cells.

Anaphylaxis A severe allergic reaction that releases histamine into the circulatory system. It occurs upon subsequent exposure to a particular antigen; also called anaphylactic shock.

Anastomosis Connecting by cross veins and forming a network.

Anasulcate Refers to pollen grains, a common form having an elongate aperture at the distal pole of the grain.

Anation Substitution of the ligand water by an anion in a coordination entity.

Anatomy The branch of morphology that deals with the structure of plants, especially the internal structure as exposed by the microscope.

Ancillary material Materials used in preparing drugs that does not become a part of the drug.

Ancipital Flattened and two-edged.

Androdioecious Having perfect and staminate flowers on separate plants, probably very rare.

Androecium Refers to the male reproductive organs of a plant.

Androgynal That bears staminate and pistillate flowers on the same parent stem.

Androgynous That has staminate and carpellate flowers in the same inflorescence.

Andromedotoxins It is a class of diterpenes causing poisoning in animals.

Androphore A stalk or tube bearing separate stamens at its apex.

Anemia Condition in which there is a reduction in the number of red blood cells or amount of hemoglobin per unit volume of blood below the standard level.

Anemo (prefix) Wind.

Anemochory Dispersal of diaspores by wind.

Anemometer A device that measures air speed.

Anemophilous Pollination by wind.

Anesthetic An herb or substance that temporarily reduces, or abolishes physical sensations. Thus it tends to eliminate pain and the sense of touch. The effect may be local or general (analgesic, anodyne, narcotic, sedative).

Aneuploid A plant with a chromosome number that is not an exact multiple of the haploid number of related plants, but is clearly similar to it.

Aneurin A vitamin that probably promotes root-growth. A growth factor for some fungi and bacteria.

Angiosperm A group of plants that produce seeds enclosed within an ovary, which may mature into a fruit. Also known as flowering plants.

Angle of divergence In a genetic spiral/parastichy, the smaller angle relative to the stem circumference separating the points of origin of two successively initiated leaves.

Angstrom A unit of length equivalent to one hundred-millionth of a centimeter (one ten-thousandth of a micron) used particularly to specify radiation wavelengths.

Angular leaf spot Bacterial blight.

Angustiseptate Refers to a fruit flattened at right angles to the septum so the septum crosses the narrowest part of the ovary.

Aniline blue Stains the cellulosic tissues.

Aniline sulphate Stains the lignified cell walls to yellow colour.

Anion A negatively charged ion.

Anion exchange resin An ion exchange material that eliminates anions from solution by exchanging them with hydroxyl ions.

Anionotropic rearrangement (or anionotropy) A type of rearrangement in which the migrating group moves with its electron pair from one atom to another.

Aniso (prefix) Unequal.

Anisocytic Type of stomata, with three subsidiary cells, two large and one smaller, surrounding the guard cells.

Anisogamy Reproduction by motile gametes that vary in morphology or behaviour.

Anisophyllous Having leaves of very dissimilar sizes and/or shapes at the same node.

Anisotropy The property of molecules and materials to show differences in physical properties along different molecular axes of the substance.

Anneal The process by which the complementary base pairs in DNA strands combine.

Annealing Refers to a treatment process for steel. The metal is heated and held at a suitable temperature and then cooled at an appropriate rate for the purpose of reducing hardness, improving machinability, facilitating cold working, producing a desired microstructure, or obtaining desired mechanical, physical, or other properties.

Annelid A segmented worm.

Annotation Adding pertinent information such as gene coded for, amino acid sequence, or other commentary to the database entry of raw sequence of DNA bases.

Annual Plant that completes its life history within a year.

Annual rings Refer to layers of wood laid down each year by the vascular cambium of woody plants, mainly in trees. Xylem cells are being added to the circumference of the xylem tissue during the season of active growth in the vascular cambium. At the beginning of the growing season, the cells grow fast and are large, but as the season progresses towards the dormant period fewer smaller cells are produced and growth finally stops as the plant becomes dormant. The difference in size of the xylem cells laid down at the start and later in the growing season forms a line within the wood marking the boundary of an annual ring. The size of the xylem cells is also affected by the growing conditions and so changes in the width of annual rings can indicate changes in the climate.

Annular Arranged in or forming a ring, annulus, a ring.

Annulation A transformation involving fusion of a new ring to a molecule via two new bonds.

Annulus In ferns, the elastic ring of more or less U-thickened cells in the sporangium wall, which initiates dehiscence.

Anode The electrode where electrons are lost (oxidized) in redox reactions.

Anodyne A herb or substance that soothes, relieves, or reduces pain without causing unconsciousness.

Anomalous Refers to a type of secondary growth that differ from the "ordinary" ones.

Anomeric effect Originally the thermodynamic preference for polar groups bonded to C-1 (the anomeric carbon of a glycopyranosyl derivative) to take up an axial position.

Anomers Diastereoisomers of glycosides, hemiacetals or related cyclic forms of sugars, or related molecules differing in configuration only at C-1 of an aldose, C-2 of a 2-ketose, etc.

Anorexia State of decreased appetite.

Anoxia Lack of oxygen or not enough oxygen.

Antacid Any substance that corrects acidity by neutralization, usually in the stomach.

Antagonist An antagonist is a drug or a compound that opposes the physiological effects of another drug.

Antagonistic muscles A pair of muscles, which work to produce opposite effects and emdash;one contracts as the other relaxes: for example, the bicep and tricep muscles on opposite sides of your upper arm.

Antenna The paired segmented sensory organs, stand one on each side of the head, commonly termed horns or feelers.

Anterior Means, in front, or toward the front.

Anthelmintic Any substance that destroys and/or expels intestinal worms.

Anther The top of the stamen, usually elevated by means of a filament, which contains the pollen.

Anther culture Refers to the culture of excised anthers on a suitable nutritive medium. Embryoids and subsequently haploid plants can be formed if anthers at a certain stage of development are taken and then cultured under appropriate condition of medium.

Antheridial cell Occurs in bryophytes and pteridophytes. A cell that develops into an atheridium.

Antheridium The organ on a gametophyte plant that produces the sperm cells.

Antherode The non-functional anther of a staminode.

Antherozoid Refers to a flagellated male gamete.

Anthesis Stage or period during which the flower bud is fully opens (flowering).

Anthocarp A true fruit surrounded by all or just the base of the perianth.

Anthochlors Chalcones.

Anthocyanidins A class of coloured anthocyanin aglycones formed from flavan-3,4-diols, also when proanthocyanidins are hydrolyzed with acid.

Anthocyanins A class of flavonoids based on the cyanidin structure, differing in the presence or absence of hydroxyl groups by methylation or glycosylation, forming colored pigments.

Anthophore A receptacular stalk bearing the corolla, androecium and gynoecium of a flower on a stalk above the height of insertion of the calyx.

Anthophyte A flowering plant, or any of its neighboring relatives, such as the Bennettitales, Gnetales, or Pentoxylales.

Anthoxanthins Any of the yellow or cream-coloured glycoside plant pigments which normally consist of a glucose molecule attached to a flavone or xanthone molecule.

Anthraquinones Quinones in which the aromatic ring is fused to both sides of a benzoquinone ring, occurring as glycosides in plants, often colored.

Antibacterial A substance with the property of killing bacteria.

Antibiotic Any substance damaging to life, but especially a substance produced by microorganism damaging or killing, other micro-organisms, or higher plants. The term is usually limited to substances of medical importance, e.g. penicillin, streptomycin, etc.

Antibiotic resistance It is the tendency of certain bacteria to develop a resistance to commonly over-used antibiotics.

Antibody A tailored protein molecule present in the blood serum or plasma (and other body fluids), whose activity is associated chiefly with gamma globulin. Produced by the immune system in response to exposure to a foreign substance, it is the body's protective mechanism against infection and disease. An antibody is characterized by a structure balancing to the foreign substance, the antigen that provokes its formation, and is thus capable of binding specifically to the foreign substance to neutralize it.

Antibody-mediated immunity Immune reaction, which protects primarily against invading viruses and bacteria through antibodies produced by plasma cells; also known as humoral immunity.

Anticlinal Those at right angles to the surface of the organ are termed as anticlinal.

Anticoagulant Any substance that prevents blood clotting, resulting in internal hemorrhaging.

Anticodon A sequence of three nucleotides on the transfer RNA molecule, which recognizes and pairs with a specific codon on a messenger RNA molecule.

Antidiabetic Any substance that helps to counteract the effects of diabetes by stabilizing blood sugar levels directly or by stimulating or mimicking the production of insulin.

Antidiarrhoeic Any substance that counteracts diarrhoea.

Antidiuretic hormone (ADH) A hormone formed by the hypothalamus and released by the pituitary gland that increases the permeability of the renal tubule of the nephron and thus increases water reabsorption. It is also known as vasopressin.

Antidote Any substance that counteracts a poison by, (a) chemically destroying the poison,

(b) mechanically preventing absorption, or (c) physiologically opposing the effects of the poison in the body after absorption.

Antidysenteric Any substance that counteracts dysentery.

Antigen Any of various foreign substances such as bacteria, viruses, endotoxins, exotoxins, foreign proteins, pollen, and vaccines, whose entry into an organism induces an immune response, i.e. antibody production, lymphokine production, or both, directed particularly against that molecule.

Antigenic determinant The site on an antigen to that an antibody binds, forming an antigen-antibody complex.

Anti-interferon An antibody to an interferon. Used for the purification of interferons.

Antihelmintic Any substance that expels or destroys intestinal worms.

Antihistamine Any substance often used in treating allergic reactions that counteracts the effect of histamine.

Antihydrotic Any substance that reduces or suppresses perspiration.

Antimicrobial Any substance that is antimicrobial possesses the property of being lethal to bacteria and other unicellular organisms.

Antinutrients Chemicals formed by plants as a defense mechanism against various factors. They inhibit the action of digestive enzymes in insects that attack and attempt to eat the plants.

Antioxidant A substance which protects tissues from damage by stabilizing harmful free radicals.

Free radicals have an unpaired electron, which is very reactive; antioxidants donate a companion electron to the free radical to 'calm it down' so that it doesn't try to react with and damage other sensitive molecules.

Antipyretic An agent that reduces or prevents fever (also called a febrifuge).

Antiraphe On the other side of the ovule to the raphe.

Anti-retroviral Any substance that acts to destroy retroviruses, RNA viruses that possess reverse transcriptase.

Antisense DNA Antisense DNA is a complementary strand of DNA that is specifically synthesized to attach to the sense DNA and prevent genetic transcription. The sense DNA that carries the information that affects the disease process is usually elucidated before an antisense drug is designed.

Antisense molecule An antisense molecule is an oligonucleotide or analog that is complementary to a segment of RNA (ribonucleic acid) or DNA (deoxyribonucleic acid) and that binds to it and inhibits its normal function.

Antiseptic Acting against sepsis. An antiseptic agent is one that has been formulated for use on living tissue to prevent or inhibit growth or action of organisms. Antiseptics should not be used to cleanse inanimate objects.

Antiserum The blood serum obtained from an animal after has been immunized with a particular antigen. It contains antibodies specific for that antigen as well as antibodies specific for any other antigens with which the animal has previously been imm-unized.

Antispasmodic Any agent that relieves spasms or cramps.

Antitoxin An antibody that is capable of neutralizing the toxin that stimulated its production in the body. Antitoxins are produced in animals for medical purposes by injection of a toxin or toxoid, with the resulting serum being used to neutralize the toxin in other individuals.

Antitropous Refers to the curva-ture of an ovule with respect to the carpel margin that bears it, curvature in the opposite direc-tion to the curvature of the margin.

Antiviral A substance that kills or inhibits the growth of viruses.

Antrorse Forward or upward.

Aorta The artery that carries blood from the left ventricle for distribution throughout the tissues of the body. It is the largest diameter and thickest walled artery in the body.

Aperients A mild and gentle acting laxative.

Aperitif An agent that stimulates the appetite.

Apert Open.

Apetalous Having flowers with-out petals or having no corolla.

Aphrodisiac Any substance that increases or arouses sexual desire, power, or potency.

API (active pharmaceutical ingredient) Also called drug substance. Any substance or mixture of substances intended to be used in the manufacture of a drug (medicinal) product and that when used in the production of a drug becomes an active ingre-dient of the drug product. Such substances are proposed to furnish pharmacological activity or other direct effect in the diagnosis, cure, mitigation, treat-ment, or prevention of disease or to affect the structure and func-tion of the body.

API starting material A material used in the production of an API which is itself or is included as a significant structural fragment into the structure of the API. A starting material may be an article of commerce, a material purchased from one or more suppliers under contract or commercial agreement, or it may be produced in-house. Starting materials are normally of defined chemical properties and structure.

Apical Refers to the tip or top of a thing.

Apical cell Refers to the upper cell formed after the first division of the zygote that further divides to produce the bulk of the embryo proper.

Apical dominance Growth of the bud at the apex of a stem or tuber while growth of all other buds on the stem or tuber is inhibited.

Apical meristem Group of cells at the growing tip of a branch or root. It divides cells to create new tissues.

Apiculate Terminated abruptly by a small, distinct point, an apiculus or apicule.

Apiculum It is a short, abrupt, flexible point (mucronate).

Apigenin It is a deoxyanthocyanin occurs in leaves and flowers.

Apnea It is a disorder in which breathing stops for periods longer than 10 seconds during sleep. It can be caused by failure of the automatic respiratory center to respond to elevated blood levels of carbon dioxide.

Apo (prefix) Separate.

Apocarpous Having separate carpels.

Apocrine glands They are sweat glands located primarily in the armpits and groin area. They are larger than the more widely distributed eccrine glands.

Apoenzyme The catalytically inactive protein portion of an enzyme that remains after removal of prosthetic group or cofactor. Examples of enzymes requiring both apoenzyme and cofactor for catalytic activity are alcohol dehydrogenase requiring Zn^{2+} kinases requiring Mg^{2+} or Mn^{2+} and cytochromes requiring Fe^{2+}.

Apogamy Development of an organism without gamete fusion (fertilization).

Apogeotropic Refers to roots which grow upwards.

Apomeiosis The division of nucleus without meiosis.

Apomixis Production of viable seed without fertilisation, equals agamospermy above, or, in a more general sense, includes the production of vegetative propagules, i.e. vegetative reproduction.

Apopetalous Polypetalous.

Apoprotein A protein without its characteristic prosthetic group or metal.

Apoptosis Means programmed cell death.

Aporphine alkaloids Group of isoquinoline alkaloids.

Apospory A kind of agamospermy where unreduced embryo sacs develop from ovular tissue.

Apothecia They are cup-shaped, spore-bearing structures produced by certain types of fungi such as Sclerotinia.

Apotracheal Axial parenchyma that is not associated with the vessels.

Apotropous Curvature of an ovule with respect to the ovary axis.

Apparent volume of distribution (V_D) Apparent volume of distribution (V_D) is the hypothetical volume of body fluid in which the drug is discovered.

Appendage It is a general term for any structure that is not one of the conventional parts of an angiosperm plant that arises from the surface of another.

Appendicular skeleton The bones of the appendages (wings, legs, and arms or fins) and of the pelvic and pectoral girdles, which join the appendages to the rest of the skeleton.

Appendix Blind sac at the end of the large intestine that frequently ruptures during final exams. It is a vestigial organ in humans.

Appetizer Any substance that excites or increases the appetite.

Apposition Term in cell wall formation, growth by deposition of layer after layer of wall material.

Appressed Lying flat or close against something.

Aquatic plants Plants that must grow in water whether rooted in the mud or floating without anchorage. It must complete part or all of their life cycle in or near the water.

Aquifer An underground layer of porous rock, sand, or gravel that contains water for wells or springs.

Arabinose An aldopentose epimeric with ribose at the 2 carbon, occurs naturally in both D- and L-forms, and is widely distributed in the form of complex polysaccharides, glycosides, and mucilages.

Arabinoside A glycoside of arabinose and occurs widely in plant species as a component of sugars.

Arachnoid Especially of hairs, looking somewhat like a spider's web.

Arborescent It is a term applied to non-woody plants attaining tree height and to shrubs tending to become tree-like in size.

Arbutin A benzoquinone.

Archaea A group of prokaryotes that can be subdivided into three groups (methanogenic, halophilic, thermoacidophilic), and are characterized by special constituents such as ether-bonded lipids and special coenzymes. They are members of a separate kingdom that falls in between eubacterial and eukaryotic organisms.

Archaebacteria Ancient, more than 3.5 billion years old, group of prokaryotes.

Archegonium It is the organ on a gametophyte plant that produces the egg cell, and nurtures the young sporophyte.

Archesporium Termed for the tissue that gives rise to megasporocytes or microsporocytes as well as parietal tissue, including the endothecium (anther) and the nucellar tissue (ovule).

Arcuate Curved like a bow.

Aril It is an often fleshy outgrowth partly or wholly covering a seed and developed from the funicle or raphe. This term is also used more generally to refer to a similar structure derived from any part of the ovule.

Aridity The condition of receiving light rainfall that is associated with cooler climates because cool air can hold less water vapor than warm air.

Arista Refers to the apex of a structure, having a stiff, bristle like awn or tip.

Aristolochic acid A phenanthrene, carboxylic acid derivative of a benzoisoquinoline precursors.

Arnaudon's green It is chromium(III) phosphate, $CrPO_4$, a green pigment.

Aromatherapy Uses essential oils extracted from medicinal plants to treat various health conditions. The oils are generally diluted, then used topically, internally, or to stimulate olfactory senses.

Aromatic A substance with a strong, volatile, fragrant aroma; frequently with stimulant properties.

Aromatic ring It is a structure found in many kinds of phytochemicals, such as phenolic compounds, alkaloids, and terpenes. It consists of six carbon atoms in a flat, hexagonal pattern. It was named so because earlier it was discovered in fragrant substances, but not all phytochemicals containing this structure have an aroma.

Aromatic waters Aromatic waters are clear, saturated aqueous solutions of volatile oils or other aromatic or volatile substances. Aromatic waters may be used as pleasantly flavored vehicles for a water-soluble drug or as an aqueous phase in an emulsion or suspension.

Arrhenius acid A substance which ionizes in aqueous solution to yield hydrogen ions (H^+).

Arteries Thick-walled vessels, which carry blood away from the heart.

Arterioles Smallest arteries and usually branched into a capillary bed.

Arteriosclerosis It is a circulatory disorder characterized by thickening and stiffening of the walls of large and medium sized arteries.

Arthritis Inflammation of the joints due to infectious, metabolic, or constitutional disorder.

Article Refers to a segment of a jointed stem, or of a fruit with constrictions between the seeds.

Articulate Having joints; jointed; provided with places where separation may take place.

Artificial selection This is the process in which breeders choose the variants to be used to create succeeding generations.

Artificially acquired active immunity This type of immunity results from immunizing an animal with a vaccine and the immunized animal produces its own antibodies and activated lymphocytes.

Artificially acquired passive immunity This type of immunity results from introducing antibodies that have been produced either in another animal or by in vitro methods into an animal. This type of immunity is only temporary.

Ascaricide Any substance that kills nematode or unsegmented worms such as roundworms and threadworms.

Ascending Rising or curving upward.

Ascidiate Refers to pitcher-shaped, more or less tubular and often widening towards a flared mouth.

Ascomycetes This is a family of fungi marked by long spore-containing cells. Forms sexual spores called ascospores, which are enclosed within a sac (a capsule structure). Ergot is an example for the same.

Ascorbate It is a mineral salt of vitamin C. They are less irritating and provide for better absorption of both vitamin C and the mineral.

Ascorbic acid It is a lactone of a sugar acid, occurs in high concentration in certain fruits and green vegetables.

Ascospores A spore produced within the sac-like cell of the sexual state of a fungus.

Ascu It is a specialized cell, characteristic of the ascomycetes, in which two haploid nuclei fuse to produce a zygote that immediately divides by meiosis. After getting matured, an ascus will contain ascospores.

Asepalous Without sepals.

Asepsis A condition in which living pathogenic (causing or capable of causing infection) organisms are absent.

Aseptic Marked by or relating to asepsis.

Aseptic processing Processing conditions designed to achieve a sterile product.

Aseptic processing area Area in which sterile product is formulated, filled into containers, and sealed.

Aseptic technique Techniques used to stop the introduction of microorganisms.

Asexual Vegetative reproduction.

Asexual reproduction A method of reproduction in that the genetically identical offspring are produced from a single parent. This occurs by many mechanisms, including fission, budding, and fragmentation.

Asperulate Slightly rough in touch.

Asphodelin It is a yellow colored anthraquinone.

Assay A technique (test) for measuring or for determining characteristics such as composition, purity, activity, and weight.

Assimilation Formation of cellular material utilizing small food molecules and energy.

Assortment A method in which meiosis produces new combinations of genetic information.

Asteotosis Refers to dry skin.

Asteototic eczema Red irritable skin resulting from severe dryness of the skin.

Aster These are short fibers produced by cells during mitosis and meiosis. These radiate from the centriole.

Asthma Disease of the respiratory tract characterized by difficult breathing, cough, and a sense of constriction in the chest.

Astringent Any substance that acts upon the albumen of organic tissues to cause condensation and contraction; it is used to decrease secretions or control bleeding. Astringents are locally applied solutions that precipitate protein.

Astrosclereid A sclereid cell with rather short, stout branches.

Asymmetric Without plane of symmetry, such that dividing the structure down its axis does not produce mirror image or identical halves.

Atactostele It is a variant of stele in which the vascular bundles are scattered through the ground tissue.

Atectate It is a pollen in which the sexine is symbolized only by isolated baculae, pilae, granules or other elements.

Atmosphere Refers to the envelope of gases that surrounds the earth. It consists largely of nitrogen (78%) and oxygen (21%).

Atom It is the smallest object that retains properties of an element. It is composed of electrons and a nucleus (containing protons and neutrons).

Atomic number Number of protons in an element.

Atomic absorption spectrophotometry A highly sensitive instrumental technique for identifying and measuring metals.

Atomic mass The average weight of an atom occurring in nature measured in atomic mass.

Atomic weight It is defined as the sum of the weights of an atom's protons and neutrons. The atomic weight differs between isotopes of the same element.

Atrioventricular (AV) node This is a tissue in the right ventricle of the heart that receives the impulse from the atria and transmits it through the ventricles by way of the bundles of His and the Purkinje fibers.

Atrioventricular (AV) valve The valve situated between each auricle and ventricle of the heart.

Atropous An erect, straight ovule with funicle, chalaza and micropyle in a straight line.

Atrophy The decrease in size or wasting of a body organ or tissue.

Attenuate Progressively narrowed to a long point at apex or base.

Aucubin It is a bitter tasting route II decarboxylated iridoid.

Auger electron spectroscopy (AES) It is an alternative surface analysis that can detect all elements with an atomic number greater than that of helium. Also it has the ability to analyze submicron-diameter features.

Aulacospermous Refers to seeds in which individual endothelial cells protrude into the endosperm and the endosperm becoming alveolate.

Aureole It is a phytoalexin.

Auricle It is a small earlike projection from the base of a leaf or petal. In animals, it refers to the chamber of the heart that receives blood from the body returned to the heart by the veins. Also known as atrium.

Aurones They are golden colored flavonoids, frequently found in flowers. They are probably formed by oxidation of chalcones.

Autapomorphic Refers to a character, derived, an evolutionary novelty of a terminal clade in a specific study, at a finer level of analysis a synapomorphy of all members of that clade.

Authentication The process of identifying.

Autochory Dispersal of diaspores without the help of any external agent.

Autoclave An apparatus into which moist heat (steam) under pressure is introduced to sterilize or decontaminate materials placed within. Steam pressure is continued for pre-specified times and then allowed to exhaust.

Autacoids It is a biological substance secreted by various cells and their physiological activity is restricted to the locality of its release. It is frequently referred to as local hormone.

Autoantibody/autoantibodies Antibodies that bind to one's own tissues rather than foreign substances. These binding results to autoimmune disease.

Autogamous Relating to, or reproducing by autogamy.

Autogamy Self-fertilization, pollination of a flower by its own pollen.

Autoimmune disorder Any condition in which the immune system reacts unsuitably to the body's own tissues and attacks them, causing damage and/or interfering with regular functioning.

Autoimmunity Autoimmunity is a tissue damaging immune response directed specifically and inappropriately against one or more self-antigens.

Automated system Any facility system or piece of equipment, which is controlled with limited or no manual intervention.

Autonomic system It is the portion of the peripheral nervous system that stimulates cardiac muscle, smooth muscle, and glands. It consists of the parasympathetic and sympathetic systems.

Autopolyploid A plant with a chromosome number that is a multiple of base number (n) of its parent, hybridisation not being involved, represented as 3X, 4X, etc.

Autoradiography A technique that uses X-ray film to visualize radioactively labeled molecules or fragments of molecules. Widely used in analyzing purposes.

Autosome A chromosome not concerned in sex determination. The diploid human genome consists of 46 chromosomes, 22 pairs of autosomes, and 1 pair of sex chromosomes.

Autotroph An organism independent of others in respect of organic nutrition, being able to fix carbon dioxide by photosynthesis, to form carbohydrates.

Autotrophic Capable of producing its own food.

Autumn wood Late wood.

Auxotroph An organism which requires a particular organic compound for growth.

Avagadro's number Number representing the number of molecules in one (1) mole: $6.023 * 10^{23}$.

Awn It is a stiff, bristle-like appendage, frequently at the end of a structure.

Axenic culture It is a culture without foreign or undesired life forms but may include the deliberate.

Axial skeleton Refers to the skull, vertebral column, and rib cage. It is one of the two components of the skeleton in vertebrates.

Axil The angle found between any two organs or structures.

Axillary In an axil, growing in an axil, as buds.

Axillary bud A bud formed in an axil.

Axis Refers to main stem or central line of growth on which secondary or side branches are borne

Axon The long part of a nerve cell that helps in the transmission of nerve impulses.

B

B cell The precursors of antibody-forming plasma cells which carry immunoglobulin and class II MHC (major histocompatibility complex) antigens on their surfaces. Also, it is a form of lymphocyte that is responsible for producing antibodies and auto-antibodies.

BAC (bacterial artificial chromosome) A vector used to clone DNA fragments in *E. coli* cells. It is based on naturally occurring F-factor plasmid found in the bacterium *E. coli*.

Baccate Form like berry.

Bacillus A rod-shaped bacterium.

Bacteria Bacteria is a general term for organisms that are composed of procaryotic cells and are not multicellular. It is the domain that contains procaryotic cells with primarily diacyl glycerol diesters in their membranes and with bacterial rRNA. Most bacteria obtain their nitrogen and energy from organic matter; some bacteria cause plant or animal diseases.

Bacterial transformation The phenomenon of incorporation of genetic material into a bacterial cell from DNA in the surrounding medium.

Bactericide An agent that kills bacteria.

Bacteriocin This is a protein produced by a bacterial strain that kills other closely related strains.

Bacteriophages Viruses that attack and kill bacterial cells.

These are composed only of DNA and protein.

Bacteriostatic Agent that inhibits growth of bacterial organisms without necessarily killing them or their spores.

Bacteriostatic water for injection It is sterile water for injection that contains one or more suitable bacteriostatic agents. It is also packaged in single or multiple dose containers of type I or II glass. These containers do not exceed the capacity of 30 mL.

Baculum In pollen, a cylindrical, free standing exine/sexine part more than 1 μm in length and less than this in diameter.

Baker's salt It is ammonium carbonate, $(NH_4)_2CO_3$.

Balanced growth Refers to microbial growth in which all cellular constituents are synthesized at constant rates relative to each other.

Balsam Refers to the resin of a tree that is healing and soothing.

Balsamum Refers to a solution of resin and volatile oil usually produced by special cells in some plants.

Band application An application in which a material such as fertilizer or herbicide is applied in strips, usually to the bed or seed row.

Barilla It is impure sodium carbonate extracted from soap-wort.

Barium white Refers to barium sulfate, $BaSO_4$.

Bark This is the outermost covering of trees and some plants.

This is composed of the cuticle or epidermis, the outer bark or cortex, and the inner bark or fiber, i.e. including phloem tissue as well as cork.

Barr body Inactivated X chromosome in mammalian females. Though inactivated, the Barr body is replicated prior to cell division and thus is passed on to all descendant cells of the embryonic cell that had one of its X chromosomes inactivated.

Barren Refers to plants not producing seed, pollen or spores capable of germination. Also plants lacking reproductive organs.

Basal body An arrangement at the base of a cilium or flagellum. It consists of nine triplet microtubules arranged in a circle with no central microtubule.

Basal cell The basal, i.e. micropylar, cells formed after the first division of the zygote, which further divides to produce the suspensor.

Basal leaves The leaves present at the base of the stem.

Base Substance which gives off hydroxide ions (OH⁻) in solution.

Base number The haploid chromosome number of the widespread ancestor of a group, represented as "x" followed by the actual number.

Base pairing The exact association between two complementary strands of nucleic acids that results from the formation of hydrogen bonds between the base components of the nucleotides of each strand: A=T and G≡C in DNA, A=U and G≡C (and in some cases G≡U) in RNA (the lines specify the number of hydrogen bonds).

Base plate The inner periclinal wall of an endothelial cell with more or less plate like and lignified thickening.

Basic Having the characteristics of a base.

Basicity It means the tendency of a compound to act as hydron (proton) acceptor. The basicity of a chemical species is usually expressed by the acidity of the conjugate acid.

Basidia Specialized club-shaped structures on the underside of club fungi, Basidiomycetes, within which spores form.

Basidiomycetes Refers to the club fungi, a major group of fungi that produce a structure (basidium) on which basidiospores are produced. Mushrooms and toadstools are included in this.

Basidiospores The spores formed on the basidia of club fungi.

Basifixed Attached at or by the base, e.g. anthers, attached by the base to the filament.

Basifugal Acropetal.

Basin Refers to a portion of a rice field bounded by levees.

Basipetal In direction from apex towards base.

Basitonic Branching particularly well developed near the base of the stem.

Bast The portion of the inner bark represented by the phloem.

Batch Refers to a specific quantity of material produced in a process or sequence of processes so that they remain homogeneous within specified limits. In case of continuous production, a batch may correspond to a defined fraction of the production, characterized by its intended homogeneity.

The size of the batch may be defined either by fixed quantity or the amount produced in a fixed time interval.

Batch number A unique grouping of numbers and/or letters that specifically identify a batch or lot and from which the production and distribution history could be determined.

Batch culture Type of culture in which microorganisms are produced by inoculating a closed culture vessel containing a single batch of medium.

Bathochromic shift (effect) Shift of a spectral band to lower frequencies (longer wavelengths) owing to the influence of substitution or a change in environment. It is casually referred to as a red shift and is opposite to hypochromic shift (blue shift).

Bay It is a part of a sea or lake indenting the shore line. This word is often applied to very large tracts of water around which the land forms a curve.

Beak It is a prominent terminal projection, especially of a carpel or fruit.

Beer-Lambert law The law describes the quantitative relationship between the absorbance of radiant energy, the concentration of the sample solution, and the length of the path through the sample.

Begonioid A leaf tooth in which there is a translucent apical pad of densely packed cells, one lateral vein strengthened at the expense of the apical and the other lateral vein, possibly close to a cucurbitoid tooth.

Behavior therapy This therapy aims at modifying behavior by reinforcing acceptable behavior and suppressing undesirable behavior.

Behcet's disease It is a complex autoimmune disease in which the body is affected by genital ulcers, mouth ulcers, eye inflammation, and several types of skin lesions.

Beneficials Refers to organisms that provide a benefit to crop production and applied especially to natural enemies of pests and to pollinators such as bees.

Benign MS A type of multiple sclerosis that is rare and mainly seen in young women. It is normally characterized by mild irregular relapses with nearly complete resolution and no disability.

Benzene An aromatic 6-carbon ring.

Benzofuran A type of terpene formed from dimethylallyl pyrophosphate and an acetate-derived polyketide precursor.

Benzoisoquinolines These are organic compounds where the benzene ring is added to an isoquinoline nucleus.

Benzoquinones Simple quinones in which an aromatic ring is fused to two oxygen atoms, there being two carbonyl groups, usually in the para (1,4) position; they are often yellow in color.

Benzylisoquinoline alkaloids A group of isoquinoline alkaloids, usually poisonous. These are modified dimers of tyrosine derived from 3.4-dihydroxytyramine (dopamine) condensed with a carbonyl compound (4:hydroxyphenylacetaldehyde), a benzene ring added to an isoquinoline nucleus.

Berberine It is a benzylisoquinoline alkaloid.

Berry Any fleshy simple fruit with one or more seeds and a skin, as a tomato, cranberry, banana, grape, etc.

Beta carotene It is a carotenoid that is stored in the liver, where the body converts it to vitamin A when required. It is found in dark, leafy greens and red, orange and yellow fruits and vegetables. Also it is a powerful antioxidant, beta carotene may play a role in slowing the progression of cancer.

Beta decay A type of radioactive decay in which a radioisotope emits a small, negatively-charged and fast-moving particle from its nucleus.

Beta-carbaline alkaloids A class of indole alkaloids that are derived from the amino acid L-tryptophan.

Betaines These are alkaloid like compound, a quaternary ammonium basic derivative.

Betalains It is a type of alkaloid, a chromalkaloid (coloured alkaloid); although not really anthocyanins, they are often called "nitrogenous anthocyanins", including betacyanins and betaxanthins.

Betaxanthins Yellow betalains.

Bi (prefix) Two, having two of anything.

Biaxial Having two axial cell rows.

Bicarbonate ions A weak base present in saliva that helps to neutralize acids in food.

Bicollateral Refers to vascular bundles with phloem on both abaxial and adaxial sides.

Biennial A plant that completes its life cycle within two years and usually does not flower until the second season.

Bifacial Refers to flattened structures, especially leaves, having distinct adaxial and abaxial surfaces.

Bifid Forked, divided by a cleft.

Biflagellate Having two flagella.

Biflavonoids A class of flavonoids, the majority of which are flavone and flavanone dimers with a simple 5, 7-4': or 5,7,3',4'-oxygenation pattern, derived from the oxidative coupling of two chalcone units and following modification of the central C3 units.

Biflavonyls A class of flavonoids produced by the dimerization of the flavone apigenin.

Bifoliolate Having two leaflets.

Biforine Cells containing raphides that have thickened, lignified walls, but usually with thin-walled papillae at the end through which raphides are quickly extruded when the side walls are deformed.

Bilateral Having two sides.

Bilaterally symmetrical Refers to corolla or calyx (or flower) when divisible into equal halves in one plane only.

Bile A digestive biochemical which emulsifies fats.

Biliary system The bile-producing system consisting of the liver, gallbladder, and associated ducts.

Bilirubin The orange-yellow pigment of bile, that aids in digestion and that is secreted by the liver. Blood tests for total bilirubin measure are performed to evaluate jaundice, anemia, various liver diseases and impaired bile excretion.

Bilocular Having two cavities.

Binary fission It is the method by which bacteria reproduce.

Binate Borne in pairs, e.g. the two leaflets of compound leaves.

Binders Binders and adhesives are added in either dry or liquid form to promote granulation or to promote cohesive compacts during direct compression.

Binding affinity It is a measure of the strength of the attraction and 'sticking power' between a protein (receptor) and its ligand (the molecule that binds to it.

Binding site A particular region or atom in a molecular unit, which is capable of entering into a stabilizing interaction with another molecular unit.

Binomial sampling The sampling method in which only the presence or absence of members of the population being sampled (such as an insect pest) on a sample unit (such as a leaf) is recorded. Does not concerns about counting the numbers of individuals.

Binomial system of nomenclature It is a system of taxonomy developed by Linnaeus in the early eighteenth century. In this system, each species of plant and animal receives a two-term name, the first term is the genus, and the second name is the species.

Binucleate Refers to the pollen grains in which the male gametophyte has two nuclei when shed from the anther.

Bioassay A procedure for determining the concentration or biological activity of a substance by measuring its effect on an organism or tissue compared with a reference standard.

Bioavailability The rate and extent at which drug is absorbed by the body when introduced in a given dosage form.

Biocatalyst It is a catalyst of biological origin, typically an enzyme.

Biochemical cycle Refers to the flow of an element through the living tissue and physical environment of an ecosystem, e.g. the carbon, hydrogen, oxygen, nitrogen, sulfur, and phosphorus cycles.

Biochemical reactions It is a specific chemical process occurring in living things.

Biochemistry Chemical processes associated with living things are called biochemistry.

Biocide An agent that kills all pathogenic and non-pathogenic living organisms, including spores. It is more general than bacteriocide.

Bioconjugates Molecular species are produced by living systems of biological origin when it is composed of two parts of different origins.

Bioconversion The change of one substance to another by biological means. One example is fermentation of sugars to alcohols, which is catalyzed by yeasts.

Biodegradable Any material that can be broken down by biological action.

Biodegradation Refers to the breaking down of a chemical by organisms in the environment.

Biodiversity It is the variety of life forms on earth. It includes genetic diversity and the concepts of species and ecological diversity as well as the ecological processes of which they are a part. The word 'biodiversity' is a short form of 'biological diversity'.

Bioequivalence Two medicines are said to be bioequivalent when they contain the same amount of an identical active moiety, and when their bioavailability is the same when administered in equal doses under equal conditions.

Bioequivalent drug products A generic drug product is considered bioequivalent to the reference (generally the brand name) drug product if both products are pharmaceutical equivalents and its rate and extent of systemic drug absorption (bioavailability) do not show a statistically significant difference when administered in the same dose of the active ingredient, in the same chemical form, in a similar dosage form, by the same route of administration, and under the same experimental conditions.

Biofix It is an identifiable event that signals when to begin degree day accumulation.

Biogeneric Biogenerics are sometimes called biosimilar products because biological products produced by different manufacturers are not strictly identical, but similar. Once approved by the regulatory board, these products are not much different in terms of quality, safety and efficacy from the originator product.

Biogeography It is the study of the distribution of plants and animals across the earth.

Biohazard An infectious agent(s), causing a real or potential risk to human, other animals, or plants, directly through infection or indirectly through disturbance of the environment.

Bioinformatics Refers to the use of computers in the life sciences, electronic databases of genomes and protein sequences, and computer modeling of biomolecules and biologic systems.

Bioisostere A bioisostere is a compound resulting from the exchange of an atom or of a group of atoms with another. The aim of a bioisosteric replacement is to create a new compound with similar biological properties to the parent compound.

Bioleaching Extraction of metals from ores or soil by biological processes, mostly by microorganisms.

Biological barrier An obstruction, either naturally occurring or introduced, to the infectivity and/or survival of a microbiological agent or eukaryotic cell once it has been released into the environment.

Biological control The action of parasites, predators, or pathogens in maintaining another organism's population bulk at a lower average level than would occur in their absence. Biological control may occur naturally or result from treatment or introduction of biological control agents by people.

Biological half life The time at which half the amount of a biomolecule in a living organism has been reduced.

Biological impurities Impurities resulting from living matter, e.g. bacteria, virus, algae, protozoa, microfungi, and their by-products, toxins.

Biological indicators To confirm that a sterilization process is effective, resistant microorganisms are placed into or on various materials. They may be placed within a filter in order to decide if a proposed autoclave cycle is effective. They are removed after autoclave, and culture tests are performed to see if the microorganisms were killed.

Biological medicinal product A medicine where the active substance is a biological substance which is produced by or extracted from a biological source.

Biology Science of life. It is concerned with the structure, function, distribution, adaptation, interactions, and evolution of all living organisms including both plants and animals.

Bioluminescent Refers to organisms that emit light under certain conditions.

Biomarker Chemical compounds that correlate with biological effects.

Biomass Refers to the material produced by the growth of microorganisms, plants or animals.

Biomembrane Biomembranes are prearranged sheet-like assemblies consisting mainly of proteins and lipids (bilayers), acting as highly selective permeability barriers, containing specific molecular pumps and gates, receptors and enzymes.

Biometabolism Refers to the physical and chemical processes that occur within a cell or an organism, e.g. the conversion of nutrients into energy.

Biomimetic Refers to a laboratory procedure designed to imitate a natural chemical process. Also refers to a compound that mimics a biological material in its structure or function.

Biomineralization The production of inorganic crystalline or amorphous mineral-like materials by living organisms. Following are few minerals synthesized biologically in various forms of life, fluoroapatite, $(Ca_5(PO_4)_3(F, OH))$, hydroxyapatite, magnetite (Fe_3O_4) and calcium carbonate $(CaCO_3)$.

Bio-pharmaceutics Bio-pharmaceutics is the study of the relation of the physical and chemical properties of a drug to its bioavailability, pharmacokinetics, and pharmacodynamic and toxicologic effects.

Biopolymers These are macromolecules (including proteins, nucleic acids and polysaccharides) formed by living organisms.

Bioprecursor prodrug A bioprecursor prodrug is a prodrug that does not imply the linkage to a carrier group, but results from a molecular modification of the active principle itself. This modification makes a new compound, which is able to be transformed metabolically or chemically, the resulting compound being the active principle.

Biopsy The gross and microscopic examination of tissues or cells for the purpose of diagnosis or prognosis of disease, or for the confirmation of normal conditions.

Bioreactor It is a closed system used for bioprocessing (flask, roller bottle, tank, vessel, or other container) that supports the growth of cells, mammalian or bacterial, in a culture medium.

Biosensor This is a device that uses specific biochemical reactions mediated by isolated enzymes, immunosystems, tissues, organelles or whole cells to detect chemical compounds, usually by electrical, thermal or optical signals.

Biosphere Refers to all ecosystems on earth as well as the earth's coating, waters, and atmosphere on and in which organisms exist. Also it refers to the sum of all living matter on earth.

Biosynthesis The production of compounds by a living organism, by biological synthesis or degradation process.

Biosynthesized A molecule is biosynthesized if it is made by living systems, opposite to laboratory synthesis.

Biotechnology Biotechnology is the study of chemical principles that support life processes. It influences drug metabolism, therapeutic effectiveness and biotransformation.

Biotic Pertains to life or living organisms.

Biotic disease Disease caused by a pathogen like bacterium, fungus, mycoplasma, or virus.

Biotransformation It is a chemical transformation mediated by living organisms or enzymes.

Biotroph Refers to parasites that derive their nutrition from the living cells of their host.

Biotype Refers to a strain of a species that has definite biological characters separating it from other individuals of that species.

Bipartite Means divided, almost to the base, into two parts.

Bipinnate Term describes a pinnate leaf in which the leaflets themselves are further subdivided in a pinnate fashion.

Birth rate Refers to the ratio between births and individuals in a specified population at a particular time.

Biseriate Set in two series or rows.

Bisexual Also known as hermaphrodite, having both female and male reproductive organs present and also functional in the same flower.

Bisporangiate Flower or cone that produces both megaspores and microspores.

Bistomal Micropyle of an ovule that is formed from both integuments.

Bisymmetric Refers to a flower, with two main planes of symmetry.

Bitter salt Refers to magnesium sulfate, $MgSO_4 \cdot 7H_2O$.

Bitter tonic Any substance that acts on the gastric mucous membranes of the mouth and stomach increasing their tone and activity and thereby improving the appetite and promoting digestion.

Black ash Impure sodium carbonate mixed with unburnt carbon (thus "black") and flame-resistant mineral residue.

Blackarm Refers to bacterial blight lesions on stems.

Bladder It is a hollow, distensible organ with muscular walls in which urine is stored and expels it through the urethra.

Bladder dysfunction Abnormal functioning of the bladder, the organ responsible for storing urine before it is eliminated from the body.

Blade Any broad and flattened region of a plant or alga, which allows for increased photosynthetic surface area (lamina).

Blank A preliminary analysis excluding only the sample to provide an unbiased reference point or baseline for comparison. In plants, nut with no kernel.

Blastocyst It is the developmental stage of the fertilized ovum by the time it is ready to implant. It is formed from the morula and consists of an inner cell mass, an internal cavity, and an outer layer of cells.

Bleaching powder It is formed by passing chlorine gas over dry calcium hydroxide, so also called chlorinated lime. When dry, the substance is mainly calcium oxychloride, $CaOCl_2$ and after absorbing moisture, it becomes a mixture of calcium chloride and hypochlorite.

Blight It is a disease characterized by common and rapid killing of leaves, flowers, and branches.

Blood-brain barrier Barrier that prevents many substances from passing out of the blood vessels to be absorbed by brain tissue.

Blood clots Formation of blood cells and fibrin strands clumped together. A clot that blocks blood flow is called a thrombus.

Blood corpuscle It is a cell that circulates in the blood.

Blood group or type It is a type of grouping into which blood can be separated on the basis of the presence or absence of certain antigens. Refers to the ABO types and the Rh blood group.

Blood plasma The resulting fluid when all blood corpuscles, with the exception of platelet cells, have been removed by centrifugation. It is a clear, straw-colored fluid, which clots as easily as whole blood.

Blood platelets These are small, disc-shaped, metabolically active cells circulating in the blood, necessary in the blood clotting process since they aggregate to form a plug on the injured surface of the blood vessel.

Blood pressure Refers to the force of the blood on the walls of arteries. Two levels of blood pressure are measured-the higher, or systolic and the lower, or diastolic, pressure. Systolic pressure occurs each time the heart pushes blood into the vessels, and the diastolic pressure occurs when the heart rests. A reading of 120/80 is said to be the normal range in which 120 is the systolic pressure and 80 is the diastolic pressure.

Blood purifier Any substance that speeds up the process of detoxification and excretion of waste products in the blood by stimulating intestinal, liver, or bile functions, or creating laxative effects.

Blood urea nitrogen (BUN) It is a waste product of the kidneys and increased levels of BUN in the blood may indicate kidney damage.

Bloom A blossom, the opening of flowers in general.

Blossom A stage or time of flowering.

Blotting This is a technique used for transferring DNA, RNA or protein from gels to a suitable binding matrix, such as nitrocellulose or nylon paper, while preserving the same physical separation.

Blue Stone It is a native crystalline copper sulfate, $CuSO_4 \cdot 5H_2O$.

BOD (biological oxygen demand) Refers to the oxygen used for metabolism of aerobic organisms in water containing organic compounds.

Body fossil The actual remains of an organism that includes bones, shells, and teeth.

Bog Referred to a marsh covered with grass or other plants. Also referred as wet or spongy ground.

Boiling point The temperature at which matter is converted from the liquid state to the gaseous state, or, the boiling point is the temperature at which the vapor pressure of a liquid equals an external pressure of 760 mm.

Bole Refers to the trunk of a tree below the lowest branch.

Bolt To start the growth of flower structures.

Bolus It is a suppository poultice used for vaginal or rectal application. It is made by mixing powdered herb material in melted cocoa butter or in a similar base. Otherwise, a mass of chewed food mixed with salivary secretions that is propelled into the esophagus during the swallowing phase of digestion.

Bond When atoms in the molecules are bonded, they are sharing one or more pairs of electrons, and maintain a particular relationship in space to one another. If one pair is shared, it's a single bond and if two pairs are shared, it is a double bond.

Bone ash It is an impure calcium phosphate.

Bone imaging The structure of bone tissue images from the radiation emitted by radionuclides that have been absorbed by the bone.

Boot Refers to a bulge in the upper leaf sheath caused by the growth of the developing panicle.

Bordeaux mixture Fungicide made of a combination of hydrated lime and copper sulfate.

Border harvesting It is a harvesting method that leaves a strip of uncut hay along every other borde. In the next harvest, these borders are trimed and the alternate borders are left standing.

Bordered Type of pit in which the pit membrane is overarched by the secondary wall, thus forming a border.

Borrow pits Depressions created on either side of a levee when soil is removed from the field to build the levee.

Botanical Refer to plants and plant life.

Bottomland Lowlands that are along streams and rivers, generally on alluvial flood plains that are periodically flooded.

Bowel dysfunction An abnormal functioning of the bowels (small and large intestines).

Brachiopods Refer to a phylum of hinge-shelled animals that have left an excellent fossil record. They live on or in the ocean floor.

Brachyparacytic Refers to paracytic stomata, with two subsidiary cells parallel to the guard cells.

Bract A modified leaf at the base of a flower.

Bracteolate These are furnished with bracteoles.

Bracteole It is a small bract, especially one on a floral axis.

Bractlet Refers either a small bract, to a floral prophyll or bracteole.

Brain imaging Brain images can be acquired by scintillation counting (scintigraphy) of radiation emitted from radioactive nuclei that have crossed the blood-brain barrier.

Brainstem Refers to the portion of the brain that is continuous with the spinal cord and consists of the medulla oblongata and pons of the hindbrain and the midbrain.

Brain The most anterior and most highly developed portion of the central nervous system.

Branch It is a natural division of a plant stem.

Branchlet Refers to a small usually terminal branch.

Bright-field microscope Refers to a microscope that illuminates the specimen directly with bright light and forms a dark image on a brighter background.

Brimstone Refers to sulfur, S.

Bristle Stiff, strong but slender hair or trichome.

Broad-spectrum drugs Refer to chemotherapeutic agents that are effective against many different kinds of pathogens.

Broad-spectrum extract An herbal extract designed to contain a wide range of the compounds found in the original plant, as opposed to a narrow spectrum extract, which focuses on achieving high levels of only one or a few compounds.

Broadcast application An application method in which a material such as fertilizer or herbicide is applied to the entire surface of a field.

Broad-spectrum pesticide Refers to a pesticide that kills a large number of unrelated species.

Brochi Refer to pollen grains, lacunae in the tectum. In animals, tubes that carry air from the trachea to the lungs.

Bronchioles Small tubes in the lungs, which are formed by the branching of the bronchi; terminate in the alveoli.

Bromcresol green $C_{21}H_{14}Br_4O_5S$, an acid-base indicator that changes from yellow to blue when the pH is raised through 5.

Bromcresol purple $C_{21}H_{16}Br_2O_5S$, an acid-base indicator that changes from yellow to purple when the pH is raised through 6.

Bromphenol blue Tetrabromophenol sulphonphthalein, $C_{19}H_{10}Br_4O_5S$, an acid-base indicator that changes color from yellow to blue when the pH rises through 3.8.

Bromphenol red Dibromophenol-sulphonphthalein, $C_{19}H_{12}Br_2O_5S$, an acid-base indicator that changes color from yellow to red when the pH rises through 6.5.

Bromthymol blue Dibromothymol-sulfonphthalein, $C_{27}H_{38}Br_2O_5S$, an acid-base indicator that changes from yellow to blue when the pH rises through 6.8.

Bronchial Any substance that relaxes constricting spasms and opens the bronchi or upper part of the lungs, thus improving respiration.

Bronchioles Refer to small tubes in the lungs that are formed by the branching of the bronchi and they terminate in the alveoli.

Bronchitis Inflammation of the bronchial mucous membranes.

Bronchodilation Refer to dilation, or opening, of the bronchial tubes.

Brood Refers to all the individuals of a generation that hatch at about the same time.

Broth Refers to the liquid culture medium in which fermentation or cell culture takes place.

Brown algae These are multicellular protistans placed in the

Division Phaeophyta that includes kelp.

Brunswick green It is a basic copper oxychloride.

Bryophyte Plants in which the gametophyte generation is the larger, persistent phase; they generally lack conducting tissues. Bryophytes include the Hepaticophyta (liverworts), Anthocerotophyta (hornworts), and Bryophyta (mosses).

Buccal and sublingual tablets Buccal and sublingual tablets allow absorption through the oral mucosa after they dissolve in the buccal pouch (buccal tablets) or below the tongue (sublingual tablets). These forms are useful for drugs that are destroyed by gastric juice or poorly absorbed from the intestinal tract.

Bud Refers to a small swelling or projection on a plant, from which a shoot, cluster of leaves, or flowers develops. Also refers to a rudimentary, undeveloped shoot, leaf, or flower.

Bud scale Refers to a scale leaf more or less surrounding a perulate resting bud.

Budding In microbiology refers to a vegetative outgrowth of yeast and some bacteria as a means of asexual reproduction; the daughter cell is smaller than the parent.

Bufadienolides They are cardiac glycosides with 6 memberd lactone ring and form C_{24} steroids. Lactone of bufadienolids has two double bonds which are attached at the 17 position of the steroidal nucleus.

Buffer A substance capable of neutralizing both acids and bases in solution, thereby maintaining the original acidity or causticity of the solution or chemicals that maintain pH values within narrow limits by absorbing or releasing hydrogen ions.

Buffer solutions Solutions that resist changes in their pH value, even when small amounts of acid or base are added.

Buffer system Pairs of weak acids and bases that maintain body fluid pH.

Bulb An underground storage organ, composed chiefly of enlarged, fleshy leaf bases.

Bulbil Refers to a small, deciduous "bulb", i.e. a rounded structure of variable construction, formed in the axil of a leaf or replacing flowers in an inflorescence, and functioning to propagate the plant vegetatively.

Bulbous Means swollen.

Bulbus Refers to the bulb or an underground bud of a plant, from which both a shoot and roots may extend.

Bulla Medical term for a skin blister.

Bulliform cells Refer to large thin-walled epidermal cells that often occur in bands down the leaf, especially in monocots.

Bundle In plants, short form for vascular bundle, often visible as a bundle scar marking the course of a vascular bundle in the outer cortex and evident when the leaf falls from the stem. Total number of bundle scars allows one to suppose the number of leaf traces and hence aspects of nodal anatomy, also bundle cap, sclerenchyma or collenchyma that forms a cap on either/both the adaxial and abaxial sides of a vascular bundle, bundle sheath, distinctive cells that entirely surround the vascular bundle.

Butter of antimony Refers to antimony trichloride, $SbCl_3$.

Butter of arsenic Refers to arsenic (III) chloride, $AsCl_3$.

Butter of tin Refers to hydrate of tin tetrachloride $SnCl_4 \cdot 5H_2O$.

Butter of zinc Refers to zinc chloride, $ZnCl_2$.

C

CADREAC Collaboration agreement between drug regulatory authorities in European Union Associated Countries (Grouping of Central and Eastern European regulatory agencies).

Caducous Refers to a plant part, such as a sepal, petal, or leaf, that falls off quickly or early.

Caespitose Growing in clumps.

Caffeic acid It is a phenol formed from cinnamic acid, more often occurs as an ester, as in chlorigenic acid.

Caffeine It is a pseudoalkaloid.

Calcareous Calcified, hardened with lime (Calcium carbonate, $CaCO_3$).

Calcareous soil Refers to soil containing high levels of calcium carbonate.

Calcification Refers to the accumulation of calcium carbonate on or in the cell walls.

Calcinosis Deposition of calcium salts into the skin, producing hard knots and sometimes ulcers.

Calcitonin Refers to a hormone produced by the thyroid, which plays a role in regulating calcium levels.

Calcium carbonate Chemical, which also occurs in limestone and marble.

Calcium oxalate They are crystals, common in plant cells, formed due to the reaction between oxalic acid of the plants and calcium from the soil.

Calibrate To standardize or correct the measuring devices on instruments.

Calibration A comparison of a standard measurement or instrument of unknown accuracy to detect, compare, report, or eliminate by adjustment of any variation in the accuracy of the unknown standard or instrument.

Callose It is a polymer of glucose.

Callus Mass of undifferentiated cells.

Calmative Any substance that produces a calming, mildly sedative, or tranquilizing effect.

Calmodulin It is a Ca^{2+} binding protein involved in metabolic regulation.

Calomel Refers to mercury(I) chloride, Hg_2Cl_2.

Calorimeter A device that measures the amount of heat in a chemical reaction.

Calorimetry An analytical method that measures heat loss or gain resulting from physical or chemical changes in a sample. Differential scanning calorimetry compares the results of heating a sample to those for heating a reference material.

Calpain It is a calcium-activated neutral protease.

Calvin cycle Sequence of biochemical, enzyme-mediated reactions during which atmospheric carbon dioxide is reduced and incorporated into organic molecules, finally some of this forms sugars. This occurs in the stroma of the chloroplast in eukaryotes.

Calycanthemous Having sepals entirely or partly converted into petals.

Calycine Pertains to the calyx.

Calyx Refers to the outer covering of a flower external to the corolla that it encloses, and consisting of a whorl of leaves, or sepals, usually of a green color and less delicate in texture than the corolla.

Calyx tube Tube formed by entirely or partially fused sepals.

CAM Refers to a photosynthetic pathway in which carbon is fixed in the dark as 4C compounds (e.g. malic acid) by phosphoenolpyruvate, these afterwards will be broken down to release CO_2 and carbon entering the plant's metabolic cycles as the 3C compound 3-phosphoglycerate.

Cambium Refers to the thin layer of undifferentiated, actively growing tissue between phloem and xylem.

Campanulate Bell-shaped, generally applied to calyx and corolla.

Campylotropous Refers to an ovule, orientated transversely with its axis at right angles to its funicle and with a curved embryo sac, the micropyle will be close to the funicle.

Canaliculate With a longitudinal groove or channel.

Cancer Refers to a group of diseases that are characterized by uncontrolled cellular growth.

Canescent More or less grey-pubescent, hoary.

Canker Refers to a dead, discolored, often sunken area (lesion) on a root, trunk, stem, or branch.

Cantharophilous Refers to plants capable of growing both in water and on land. Also, growing with part of the plant in the water or mud and part in the air

Capillaries Refer to small, thin-walled blood vessels that allow oxygen to diffuse from the blood into the cells and carbon dioxide to diffuse from the cells into the blood.

Capillary bed A branching network of capillaries supplied by arterioles and drained by venules.

Capitate Shaped like a head, swollen at one or both ends

Capping Capping is the partial or complete separation of the top or bottom crown from the main body of the tablet.

Capsid Refers to the external protein shell or coat of a virus particle.

Capsule Refers usually to a dry fruit formed from two or more united carpels and dehiscing at maturity to release the seeds, sometimes with valves (or) capsules are solid dosage forms in which one or more medicinal or inert substances are enclosed within a small gelatin shell. Gelatin capsules may be hard or soft.

Carbanion Refers to the generic name for anions containing an even number of electrons and having an unshared pair of electrons on a tervalent carbon atom.

Carbene Generic name for the species H_2C: and substitution derivatives thereof, containing an electrically neutral bivalent carbon atom with two nonbonding electrons.

Carbocation Refers to a cation containing an even number of electrons with a significant portion of the excess positive charge situated on one or more carbon atoms.

Carbohydrates A large class of carbon-hydrogen-oxygen compounds that includes the sugars and their polymers (mainly starch, glycogen and cellulose). Most carbohydrates are produced by photosynthesis in plants. They are the major food compounds for both plants and animals.

Carbon cycle Describes the pathway of movement of carbon ecosystem, i.e. from one component to other component of ecosystem that included in both living organisms and abiotic environment.

Carbon filter A vessel loaded with activated carbon that is used to remove organics, chlorine, tastes, and odors from liquids, operating on the principle of adsorption.

Carbon monoxide dehydrogenases Enzymes which catalyze the oxidation of carbon monoxide to carbon dioxide.

Carbonate hardness Refers to the hardness in water caused by bicarbonates and carbonates of calcium and magnesium. If alkalinity goes beyond total hardness, all hardness is carbonate hardness; if hardness goes beyond alkalinity, the carbonate hardness equals the alkalinity.

Carbonic anhydrase It is a zinc-containing enzyme that catalyzes the reversible decomposition of carbonic acid to carbon dioxide and water.

Carboxylated iridoids It is a kind of route II iridoid derived from epi-iridodial and epi-iridotrial through glucosylation and oxidation of C_{11} to the carboxyl level.

Carboxylic acids Carboxylic acids have a general formula of R – COOH and contain a carboxyl group (-COOH).

Carcinogen Refers to a substance that causes the development of cancerous growths in living tissue.

Carcinogenic Cancer-causing. Many agents that are carcinogenic are mutagens.

Carcinostatic Any substance that arrests or inhibits the development or continued growth of cancer, carcinomas, or malignant tumors.

Cardenolides They are cardiac glycosides having an unsaturated butyrolactone ring and form a C_{23} steroids. The lactone of cardenolides has a single double bond and is attached at the C-17 position of steroidal nucleus.

Cardiac cycle Refers to one heartbeat. It consists of atrial contraction and relaxation, ventricular contraction and relaxation, and a short pause.

Cardiac glycosides A type of cardenolide.

Cardiac muscle The type of muscle that is found in the walls of the heart.

Cardiac tonic Any substance, or combined formula that strengthens and stimulates the heart metabolism.

Cardialgic Any substance that causes heartburn.

Cardiovascular system The human circulatory system consisting of the heart and the vessels, which transport blood to and from the heart.

Carinate Shaped like the keel of a ship, having a longitudinal prominence on the back, like a keel, mainly refers to a calyx, corolla or leaf.

Carminative Any substance that aids, prevents, or relieves the expelling of gas and flatulence from the stomach, intestines, and/or bowels, and thus reduces pain and discomfort.

Carnivores Term applied to a heterotroph, usually an animal, that eats other animals.

Carotenoids Refer to subclass of fat-soluble terpenes that consist of two diterpene phytol-like units (C_{40} compounds, 8 isoprene units).

Carpals Refers to the bones that make up the wrist joint.

Carpel A simple pistil, regarded as a modified leaf; also, any of the two or more carpels that unite to form a compound pistil. It is the unit of structure of the female portion of a flower.

Carpellate With functional carpels only.

Carpellode Refers to a non-functional carpel.

Carpidiophore Refers to a persistent woody fruit base of a capsule or schizocarp.

Carpophore Refers to the central axis that persists between the carpels in a schizocarp where the ovary is inferior.

Carrier Any substance that is added to a formula or mixture of other herbs to aid in the distribution of the medicine to the proper location in the body or to enhance the effect of the other principle ingredients. In microbiology, an infected individual who is a potential source of infection for others and plays an important role in the epidemiology of a disease.

Carrier-linked prodrug It is a prodrug that contains a temporary linkage of a given active substance with a temporary carrier group, which produces improved physicochemical or pharmacokinetic properties and that can be easily removed in vivo.

Cartilaginous Fleshy, but firm or even hard and leathery.

Caruncle Refers to a more or less plump excrescent outgrowth from the surface of a seed, usually near the hilum or micropyle.

Caryophyllaceous Refers to diacytic (of stomata).

Caryopsis Refers to a small one seeded, dry, indehiscent fruit, seeds adhering to the thin pericarp, thus the fruit and seed are incorporated into one body, as in wheat and other kinds of grain.

Cascade prodrug Refers to a prodrug for which the cleavage of the carrier group becomes effective only after unmasking an activating group.

Casparian band Refers to a waxy band-like formation within primary walls that contains lignin and suberin situated in the anticlinal walls, especially in endodermis or an impermeable waxy layer between the cells of the endodermis, which stops water and solutes from entering the xylem, except by passing through the cytoplasm of adjacent cells.

Castanospermine It is a polyhydroxy alkaloid.

Casuarinine It is a polyhydroxy alkaloid.

CAT scan Acronym for computerized axial tomography. It is a test used to view internal body structures and also known as CT scan.

Cata Refers to the apertures of pollen grains, situated at or towards the proximal pole, a very rare arrangement.

Catabolic reactions Reactions in cells in which existing chemical bonds are broken and molecules are broken down.

Catabolism The intracellular phase of metabolism involved in the energy-yielding degradation of nutrient molecules (e.g. glucose to CO_2 and H_2O) and the waste products are called catabolites.

Catalase It is an enzyme that catalyzes the decomposition of hydrogen peroxide into oxygen and water.

Catalyst Refers to a compound that increases the rate of a chemical reaction without being consumed or changed. In the biosciences, the term enzyme is used and enzymes catalyze biological reactions.

Cataphyll Refers to any rudimentary leaf, as a bud scale, prior to the true foliage leaves.

Catarrh Refers to inflammation of a mucous membrane, particularly of the respiratory tract.

Caterpillar The larva of a butterfly, moth, sawfly, or scorpionfly.

Cathartic Any substance that has a strong laxative effect that causes or hastens an evacuation of the bowels.

Cathode Refers to electrode where electrons are gained (reduction) in redox reactions.

Cation It is a positively charged particle or ion.

Cation exchange The displacement of one positively charged particle by another on a cation-exchange material.

Cation exchange resin It is an Ion exchange resin that removes positively charged ions (cations) by exchanging them for hydrogen ions.

Catkin Refers to a spike-like cluster of unisexual flowers.

Cauda A process resembles tail.

Caudate Refers to an appendage at the apex of a leaf.

Cauline Refers to leaves, borne on an aerial stem, generally separated by elongated internodes.

Caulome A collective term for all stems of a plant and their modifications.

Caustic Any substance that contains acidic material that has an escharotic or corrosive action capable of burning or eating away living tissues.

CBC An acronym for "complete blood count".

Cecidium Gall.

Cell It is the basic building block of human tissues. Cells work jointly to produce tissues within the body. Different tissues working together produce functional organs such as the kidney, heart, brain, and skin.

Cell body In a neuron, it refers to the part that contains the nucleus and most of the cytoplasm and the organelles.

Cell culture The in vitro propagation of cells removed from organisms in a laboratory environment that has strict sterility, temperature, and nutrient requirement.

Cell cycle The sequence of events from one division of a cell to the next.

Cell differentiation It is the process whereby offsprings of a common parental cell achieve and maintain specialization of structure and function. Muscle cells become muscle cells and bone cells start to develop. In humans, all the different types of cells differentiate from the simple sperm and egg.

Cell fusion Fusion of two or more cells to become a single cell.

Cell generation time The interval between consecutive divisions of a cell.

Cell line Cells that begin from a primary culture at the time of the first successful subculture.

Cell-mediated immunity Type of immunity that results from T cells coming into close contact with foreign cells or infected cells to destroy them. Also it can be transferred to a nonimmune individual by the transfer of cells.

Cell plate In plants, it refers to a membrane-bound space produced during cytokinesis by the vesicles of the Golgi apparatus. The cell plate fuses with the plasma membrane thereby dividing the cell into two compartments.

Cell theory The cell theory states that all living things are composed of at least one cell and also states that the cell is the fundamental unit of function in all organisms.

Cell wall Structure produced by some cells outside their cell membrane. It is composed of chitin, peptidoglycan, or cellulose.

Cellular Refers to endosperm formation, where all nuclear divisions of the endosperm are accompanied by cell wall formation.

Cellular respiration The transfer of energy from various molecules to produce ATP. It occurs in the mitochondria of eukaryotes and the cytoplasm of prokaryotes. In this process, oxygen is consumed and carbon dioxide is generated.

Cellulase It is an enzyme that is capable of digesting cellulose into simpler units.

Cellulitis It is a pattern of inflammation of the skin resulting from infection with bacteria.

Cellulose The chief substance composing the cell walls or woody part of plants. It is a carbohydrate of unknown molecular structure but having the composition represented by the empirical formula $(C_6H_{10}O_5)_x$.

Celsius Pertains to a temperature scale that records the freezing point of water as 0°C and the boiling point as 100°C under normal atmospheric pressure. It is also called centigrade.

Central nervous system (CNS) The division of the nervous system which, includes the brain, spinal cord, and brainstem, along with other structures.

Centrifugal Developing from the center outward.

Centrifugation It is a mechanical means of separation based on differences in sedimentation rates due to differences in density between the suspended particles in the liquid.

Centrifuge A centrifuge functions on the principle of centrifugal force, the inertial reaction by which a body tends to move away from a center about which it revolves. This is commonly used to separate solids from liquids or liquids of dissimilar densities.

Centripetal That develops inward toward the center.

Centriole Paired cellular organelle that functions in the organization of the mitotic spindle during cell division in eukaryotes.

Centromere Refers to the site on the chromosome where spindle fibers attach during nuclear division.

Ceratolin It is a dihydrochalcone.

Cerebellum Part of the brain concerned with fine motor coordination and body movement, posture, and balance.

Cerebral cortex The outer layer of gray matter in the cerebrum which, consists mainly of neuronal cell bodies and dendrites in humans. It is associated with higher functions, including language and abstract thought.

Cerebrum The part of the forebrain that includes the cerebral cortex also it is the largest part of the human brain.

Certified seed Refers to seeds, tubers or young plants certified by a recognized authority to be free of or to contain less than a minimum number of specified pests or pathogens.

Ceruloplasmin It is a copper protein present in blood plasma.

Cervix Refers to the lower neck of the uterus that opens into the vagina.

CGMPS (current good manufacturing practices) Current accepted standards of design, operation, practice and sanitization.

Chaff Refers to dry scales or bracts, as those on the receptacle subtending the flowers in the heads of certain plants.

Chaffy Refers to texture, thin and membranous.

Chain reaction It is a reaction in which one or more reactive reaction intermediates are continu-

ously regenerated, usually through a repetitive cycle of elementary steps.

Chakras The seven vital energy centers of the body that extend from the base of spine to the crown of head. It is located in the rectal area, near the genitals, behind the navel, at the heart, at the neck, between the eyebrows, and on the crown of the head. Each chakra corresponds to certain colors, emotions, organs, nerve networks, and energies.

Chalaza Part of an ovule to which the end of the funicle is attached and below the insertion of the integuments.

Chalazogamy Process of fertilisation during which the pollen tube penetrates the ovule by way of the chalaza.

Chalazosperm Refers to nutritive tissue in a seed, developed from persistent chalazal cells.

Chalcones Flavonoids isomeric with flavanones, often yellow, but turning orange red in the presence of ammonia.

Channeled Having a deep longitudinal groove.

Channels Refer to transport proteins that act as gates to control the movement of sodium and potassium ions across the plasma membrane of a nerve cell.

Chaperonin Member of the set of molecular chaperones, located in different organelles of the cell and involved either in transport of proteins through biomembranes by unfolding and refolding the proteins or in assembling newly formed polypeptides.

Character Refers to any feature of the organism.

Characterization Accurately reading and describing all the characteristics of a drug substance that affect its efficacy and its purity. Also referes to the chemical, physical, and sometimes biological properties that are attributes of a specific drug substance.

Charcoal Either a charred carbonaceous material or its primary constituent, namely carbon.

Charge Explains an object's ability to repel or attract other objects. Protons have positive charges while electrons have negative charges.

Chartaceous Papery in texture.

Chelation Chelation involves coordination of more than one sigma-electron pair donor group from the same ligand to the same central atom.

Chelation therapy Chelation therapy is a series of intravenous injections of the synthetic amino acid EDTA, designed to detoxify the body. Frequently used to treat arteriosclerosis, angina, Alzheimer's disease.

Chelating agents Refer to organic compounds that can withdraw ions from solution, forming insoluble complexes.

Chelidonic acid It is an organic acid derived from a condensation of C_3 and C_4 units related to phosphoenolpyruvic acid and erythrose-4-phosphate.

Chemical reaction A process that results in the interconversion of chemical species. It may be elementary reactions or stepwise reactions.

Chemical species That have chemically identical things.

Chemically defined medium A nutritive solution or substrate for culturing cells.

Chemiosmosis It is the process by which ATP is produced in the inner membrane of a mitochondrion.

Chemoautotrophs Facultative autotrophs that obtain their energy from the oxidation of inorganic compounds.

Chemoselective Chemoselectivity is the preferential reaction of a chemical reagent with one of two or more different functional groups.

Chemostat It is a growth chamber that keeps a bacterial culture at a specific volume and rate of growth by limiting nutrient medium and removing spent culture.

Chemotaxis Used for describing principles and practices of classification of plants on the basis of chemical analysis.

Chemotherapy Treatment of disease by means of chemical substances or drugs.

Chemotrophs Organisms, generally bacteria, which derive energy from inorganic reactions; also known as chemosynthetic.

Chewable tablets Chewable tablets disintegrate smoothly and rapidly when chewed or allowed to dissolve in the mouth.

Chimera A recombinant plasmid containing foreign DNA that is used as a cloning vector in genetic engineering.

Chiral Having the property of chirality.

Chirality A term describing the geometric property of a rigid object that is non-superimposable on its mirror image; such an object has no symmetry elements of the second kind.

Chirality centre Refers to an atom holding a set of ligands in a spatial arrangement which is not superposable on its mirror image.

Chirality plane A planar unit connected to an neighboring part of the structure by a bond which results in restricted torsion so that the plane cannot lie in a symmetry plane.

Chirality sense Refers to the property that distinguishes enantiomorphs.

Chitin A polysaccharide contained in fungi; also forms part of the hard outer covering of insects.

Chlorinated vinyls Thermoplastic chlorinated vinyls comprise PVC, CPVC, and VDC. PVC and CPVC are very similar materials, the main difference being the addition of more chlorine to the PVC molecule to synthesize CPVC. This results in a higher glass transition temperature that equates to a higher use temperature for CPVC.

Chlorination Addition of chlorine or chlorine compounds to water for disinfection.

Chlorine Chemical used to kill microorganisms in water. A greenish yellow gas at room temperature and atmospheric pressure.

Chlorofluorocarbons (CFCs) Chemical substances that are used in refrigerators, air conditioners, and solvents that drift to the upper stratosphere and dissociate.

Chlorogenic acid Type of phenylpropanoid.

Chlorophyll Photosynthetic pigment common to all photosynthetic organisms (green plants or green).

Chlorophylla The green photosynthetic pigment, which is common to all photosynthetic organisms.

Chlorophyll b An accessory chlorophyll that is found in green algae and plants.

Chlorophyll c An accessory chlorophyll that is found in some protistans.

Chlorophyta The taxonomic division, which contains what are commonly called the green algae.

Chloroplasts They are relatively large, chlorophyll containing, green organelles responsible for photosynthesis in photosynthetic eukaryotes, such as algae and plant cells.

Chlorosis It is an abnormal condition characterized by absence of green pigments in plants.

Cholecystokinin Refers to a hormone secreted in the duodenum, which causes the gallbladder to release bile and the pancreas to secrete lipase.

Cholegogue An agent that stimulates secretion and release of bile.

Cholera A bacterial disease contracted through contaminated drinking water. Its symptoms include severe gastrointestinal problems such as acute diarrhea and infection of the small intestine.

Choleretic Agent that stimulates the formation of bile.

Cholesterol An important component of blood lipids (fats) manufactured by the liver that's also the precursor of the steroid hormones, such as the sex and "fight or flight" hormones. Few types, specifically low-density lipoprotein (LDL) and very-low-density lipoprotein (VLDL), if oxidized, can collect inside artery walls as plaque, restricting blood flow, reducing vessel flexibility and leading to heart disease. High-density lipoprotein (HDL) helps move LDL cholesterol out of the system.

Chorion The outer membrane of an insect egg.

Choripetalous Having unconnected or separate petals.

Chorisepalous Polysepalous.

Chromatids Refers to copies of a chromosome produced by replication.

Chromatin The complex of DNA and protein in the nucleus of the interphase cell, originally recognized by its reaction with stains specific for DNA.

Chromatography The word is made up of Greek roots meaning 'chromas-color' and 'graphy-writing'. It is an analytical technique for resolution of solutes, in which separation is made by differential migration in a porous medium and migration is caused by flow of solvent or gas.

Chromoalkaloids Refers to betalains.

Chromogen A colorless substrate that is acted on by an enzyme to produce a colored end product.

Chromones A type of coumarin consisting of a benzene ring fused to a pyrone ring with a methyl group at the C_2 position and oxygenated at the C_5 and C_7 positions.

Chromophore Refers to the part of a molecular entity consisting

of an atom or group of atoms in which the electronic transition responsible for a given spectral band is approximately localized.

Chromoplast A plastid with abundant yellow or orange carotenoids.

Chromosome A thread-like structure in the nucleus or chloroplasts of a cell, containing a linear sequence of genes.

Chromosome theory of inheritance States that chromosomes are the cellular components that physically contain genes that is proposed in 1903 by Walter Sutton and Theodore Boveri.

Chronic A condition that often lasts a long duration and is slow in progress; not acute.

Chrysophanol An anthraquinone.

Chrysophytes Protistan division, which is referred to as the golden brown algae, includes the diatoms.

Cilia Refers to hair-like organelles extending from the membrane of many eukaryotic cells; often function in locomotion.

Ciliata With marginal hairs that form a fringe.

Cinereous Refers to ash-grey, as of wood ash.

Cinnamic acid A simple phenol derived from L-phenylalanine, involved in formation of phenylpropanoids, occurring in various aromatic resins.

Circulative virus A virus that systemically infects its insect vector and usually is transmitted for the remainder of the vector's life.

Circulatory system One of eleven major body organ systems in animals, which transports oxygen, carbon dioxide, nutrients, and waste products between cells and the respiratory system and carries chemical signals from the endocrine system. It consists of the blood, heart, and blood vessels.

Circulatory system, closed System that uses a continuous series of vessels of different sizes to deliver blood to body cells and return it to the heart that is found in echinoderms and vertebrates.

Circulatory system, open System in which the circulating fluid is not enclosed in vessels at all times that is found in insects, crayfish, some mollusks, and other invertebrates.

Circumscissile Splitting by a transverse fissure around the circumference, leaving an upper and lower half. Refers to certain seed pods or capsules.

Cis, trans The two ligands are said to be located *cis* to each other if they lie on the same side of a plane. If they are on opposite sides, their relative position is described as *trans*.

Cladode A photosynthetic stem of a plant whose foliage leaves are absent or much reduced.

Cladophyll Refers to phylloclade.

Cladoptosis Loss of whole branches or branchlets by abscission at the base.

Class A grade in the taxonomic hierarchy with the termination – ales or taxonomic subcategories of phyla.

Classic dermatomyositis Patients having the hallmark cutaneous manifestations of dermatomyositis, proximal muscle weakness, and objective evidence of muscle inflammation characteristic of dermatomyositis.

Clathrate Latticed or pierced with apertures like a trellis.

Clavate Refers to club-shaped, rather gradually widening towards the apex.

Claw A sharply narrowed and stalk-like basal portion of a petal, sepal or bract.

Clay Refers to the soil particles derived from weathering of mineral rock during soil formation and having size less than 0.002 mm and consists of alumino-silicates in a latticed structure.

Clearance Clearance is the volume of plasma cleared of drug per unit time.

Cleft That is divided halfway down to the midrib or further, or generally, any deep lobe or cut.

Clinical pharmacokinetics Clinical pharmacokinetics is the application of pharmacokinetic principles for the rational design of an individualized dosage regimen. The two main objectives are maintenance of an optimum drug concentration at the receptor site to produce the desired therapeutic response for a specific period and minimization of any adverse or toxic effects of the drug.

Clinical trials Testing of INDs (investigational new drugs) in human subjects to prove safety and efficacy prior to the drug's approval for marketing. The investigation is generally divided into three phases for a untested drug: Phase I: Introducing the drug into a small number, generally 20 to 80, patients or healthy volunteers to determine the drug's metabolism, pharmacological actions, and side effects associated with increasing doses. Phase II: introducing the drug into a small number, generally no more than several hundred, patients with the disease to evaluate the effectiveness of the drug, common short-term side effects and risks associated with its use. Phase III: Introducing the drug into several hundred to several thousand subjects. Studies are expanded controlled and uncontrolled trials performed after preliminary evidence suggesting effectiveness of the drug has been obtained. If the results of the phase III clinical trials are favorable, then the FDA will normally license the drug for manufacture and sale.

Clockwise Of plants, the direction of twining, the stem taking an ascending clockwise course when viewed from above.

Clonal propagation Asexual multiplication of plants from a single entity or explant.

Clone A population asexually derived from a single cell or individual.

Cloning A specialized DNA technology to produce multiple, exact copies of a single gene or other segment of DNA to obtain enough material for further study. This process is used by researchers in the human genome project, and is referred to as cloning DNA.

Cloning vector DNA molecule originating from a virus, a plasmid, or the cell of a higher organism into which another DNA fragment of suitable size can be integrated without loss of the vectors capacity for self-replication; vectors introduce foreign DNA into host cells, where it can be reproduced in big quantities. Examples are plasmids, cosmids, and yeast artificial chromosomes.

Closed meristem Refers to root apical meristem in which one or more tissue regions of the root can be traced to separate initials.

Clostridium Genus of bacteria, most are obligate anaerobes that form endospores.

Coagulation Adding insoluble compounds to water to neutralize the electrical charge on colloids, causing them to coalesce to form larger particles that can be removed by settling.

Coaguligand Refers to a VTA (vascular targeting agent) that utilizes a human coagulation protein to induce tumor blood vessel clotting.

Coalescence Coalescence occurs in emulsion systems when the liquid particles of the dispersed phase merge to form larger particles. Coalescence is largely prevented by the interfacial film of surfactant around the droplets.

Cobalamin Vitamin B_{12}.

Cobweb Formed of tangled hairs or fibres.

Cocarcinogenins Refers to phorbol ester diterpenes, which is a type of carcinogen that promotes neoplastic growth only after its initiation by another substance.

Coccus A bacterium of round, spheroidal, or ovoid form, including Micrococcus, Staphylococcus, Streptococcus, and Pneumococcus (or) in plants mericarp.

Coding sequence Refers to the region of a gene (DNA) that encodes the amino acid sequence of a protein.

Codon A sequence of three consecutive nucleotides that occurs in mRNA and directs the inclusion of a specific amino acid into a protein, or symbolizes the starting or termination signal of protein synthesis.

Coenocyte A cell in which the nuclei divide, but not the cytoplasm that results in a cell containing several nuclei.

Coenzyme Refers to a non-polypeptide molecule required for the action of certain enzymes; frequently contains a vitamin as a component. [Coenzyme I (diphosphopyridine nucleotide) Coenzyme II (triphosphopyridine nucleotide)].

Coenzyme A A coenzyme that is necessary for the oxidative decarboxylation of pyruvates.

Coenzyme Q (ubiquinone) Used for a lipid soluble electron carrying coenzyme which takes part in transport of electron from NAD to oxygen in the respiratory chain. Molecule is a reversibly reducible quinone.

Cofactor Small molecular weight, heat stable inorganic or organic substance required for the action of an enzyme.

Coflorescence The cluster of flowers that terminates a lateral branch of a synflorescence.

Cognition Functions carried out by the brain, some of which include memory, planning, problem-solving, construction, calculation, and attention.

Coherent Having parts united.

Colchicine $C_{22}H_{25}O_6N$. An alkaloid drug which is extracted from the corm of the autumn crocus *Colchicum autumnale*. It causes abnormal division of nuclei, resulting in an increase of the chromosome number forming a polyploid.

Cole crops Any of the group of crucifer family.

Coleoptile A tubular structure developed at the junction of the cotyledonary sheath and surrounding the plumule of a monocot embryo or seedling.

Colic Disease characterized by severe pain in the gut due to various affections of the gastrointestinal tract.

Coliform bacteria A group of bacteria found in mammalian intestines and soil, used as a measure of fecal pollution in water. They are easy to identify and count in the laboratory because of their ability to ferment lactose.

Collagen An albuminoid present in connective tissue, bone (ossein), and cartilage (chondrin), notable for its high content of the imino acids proline and hydroproxilone. On boiling with water, it is converted into gelatin.

Collar Region of junction between blade and leaf sheath of grasses.

Collateral Of buds, ovules, situated side by side, and therefore not on the same radius.

Collateral targeting The therapeutic strategy of targeting structures and cell types other than cancer cells common to all solid tumors as a means to attack a solid tumor.

Collective fruit A single fruit which is formed from several flowers.

Collenchyma Living, supportive tissue with chloroplasts generally just beneath the surface consisting or more or less elongated cells usually thickened unevenly in a manner somewhat variable in different groups of plants.

Colligation The formation of a covalent bond by the combination or recombination of two radicals.

Colligative properties Properties of a solution that depend only on the number of particles dissolved in it, not the properties of the particles themselves.

Colloids Fine particles they will not settle without prior coagulation. They range from 10 Å to 1,000 Å (Angstroms).

Colon hydrotherapy Cleansing the large intestine with warm purified water. A single colonic treatment is said to be equivalent to several enemas in removing toxic debris from the colon.

Colonoscopy Examination of the colon through a flexible, lighted instrument called a colonoscope.

Colony A growth of microorganisms on a solid medium. The growth is visible without magnification.

Colony-stimulating factors Colony-stimulating factors (CSFs) are a class of glycoprotein hormones. CSFs regulate the differentiation and formation of blood cells from precursor cells.

Colony forming unit (CFU) Measuring the number of bacteria present in the environment or on the surfaces of an aseptic processing room that is measured as part of qualification and ongoing monitoring. An indication of the number of viable microorganisms in a sample.

Columella A small column of tissue which runs up through the center of a spore capsule.

Coma A sleep-like state; unconscious. May be due to a high or low level of glucose (sugar) in the blood.

Comatose In a coma, unconscious.

Comb Deeply divided with the segments narrow and close.

Combinatorial biology Introduction of genes from one microorganism into another microorganism to synthesize a new product or a modified product, particularly in relation to antibiotic synthesis.

Combinatorial library It is a set of compounds prepared by combinatorial synthesis.

Combinatorial synthesis It is a process to prepare large sets of organic compounds by combining sets of building blocks.

Combustible dust Refers to any finely divided solid material that is 420 μ or less in diameter, or any material capable of passing through an US no. 40 standard sieve that when dispersed in air in the proper proportions, could be ignited by a flame, spark or other source of ignition.

Combustible liquid Refers to any liquid having a closed cup flash point at or above 100°F (37.8°C). They do not include compressed gases or cryogenic fluids.

Combustion When substances combine with oxygen and release energy.

Commissure Of plants, as where one carpel joins another in the Umbelliferae.

Common cold An acute, self-limiting, and highly contagious virus infection of the upper respiratory tract that produces inflammation, profuse discharge, and other symptoms.

Common symptoms Symptoms that are common to a specific disease (yellow skin in jaundice).

Communicable disease A disease associated with a pathogen that can be transmitted from one host to another.

Companion cells Specialized cells in the phloem that load sugars into the sieve elements and help maintain a functional plasma membrane in the sieve elements.

Complementary DNA A DNA copy of an RNA molecule.

Complementary medicine Any type of therapy used in combination with other alternative treatments or standard/conventional medicine.

Complementary nucleotides The bonding preferences of nucleotides, adenine with thymine, and cytosine with guanine.

Complementary sequence Nucleic acid-base sequence that can form a double stranded structure by matching base pairs with another sequence; the complementary sequence to GTAC is CATG.

Complement system A chemical defense system, which kills microorganisms directly, supplements the inflammatory response, and works with, or complements, the immune system.

Complete blood count (CBC) A counting of the number of red blood cells, white blood cells, and platelets that are circulating in the blood.

Complex medium Any culture medium that contains some ingredients of unknown chemical composition.

Complete flower Flower in which all flower parts are present.

Compound fruit A fruit that is made up of two or more distinct carpels.

Compound leaf A leaf having two or more distinct leaflets that

are evident as such from early in development.

Compound Refers to a chemical composed of more than one type of atom, e.g. sulfur (S) is an element, but allicin is a compound containing sulfur, oxygen, carbon and hydrogen.

Compounding Bringing together of excipient and solvent components into a homogeneous mix of active ingredients.

Compounding pharmacy An old fashion type of pharmacy that still mixes medications to doctors specifications such as pouring prescribed amounts of drug powder into capsules.

Compressed Flattened in one plane, either dorsally or laterally.

Compressed gas Any material, or mixture of materials that are either liquefied, nonliquefied, or in solution having a boiling point of 68°F (20°C) or less at 14.7 psia (101.3 kpa) of pressure.

Compressed tablets Compressed tablets are formed by compression and have no special coating. They are made from powdered, crystalline, or granular materials, alone or in combination with excipients such as binders, disintegrants, diluents, and colorant's.

Computational chemistry It is a discipline using mathematical methods for the calculation of molecular properties or for the simulation of molecular behaviour.

Computer-assisted drug design (CADD) Computer-assisted drug design involves all computer-assisted techniques used to discover, design and optimize bioactive compounds with a supposed use as drugs.

Concanavalin A It is a protein from jack beans, containing calcium and manganese, which agglutinates red blood cells and stimulates T lymphocytes to undergo mitosis.

Concave Refers to surface that curves inward.

Concentration The amount of substance in a specified space.

Concretion The act or process of making or becoming solid.

Concurrent process validation Establishing documented evidence that a process does what it claims to do based on information generated during actual implementation of the process.

Condensate Refers to distillate just after it has been cooled from steam into the liquid state.

Condensation reaction A (typically stepwise) reaction in which two or more reactants (or remote reactive sites within the same molecular entity) yield a single main product with accompanying formation of water or of some other small molecule.

Condenser The heat exchanger used in distillation unit to cool steam in order to convert it from the vapor to the liquid state.

Condensed tannins Proanthocyanidins.

Condiment Enhances the flavor of food.

Conduction Movement or transmission of a nerve impulse.

Condyle Inward projection of the endocarp around which the seed is folded.

Cone In conifers, a compact group of reduced branches to which the ovules are attached.

Conformation The spacial arrangements of atoms affording distinction between stereoisomers that can be interconverted by rotations about formally single bonds.

Conformational analysis The assessment of the relative energies, reactivities, and physical properties of alternative conformations of a molecular entity, typically by the application of qualitative or semi-quantitative rules or by semi-empirical calculations.

Conformer One of a set of *stereoisomers*, each of that is characterised by a *conformation* corresponding to a different potential energy minimum.

Congener A congener is a substance literally con- (with) generated or synthesized by essentially the same synthetic chemical reactions and the same procedures.

Congenital Refers to fusion of parts from the very beginning of development.

Congested Densely crowded.

Conidium Type of asexual fungal spore.

Conifers Group of gymnosperms that reproduce by cones and have needle-like leaves, includes the pines.

Coniine A pyridine alkaloid.

Conjugated protein A protein containing a metal or an organic prosthetic group or both, e.g. hemoglobin.

Conjugate acid A substance which can lose an H^+ ion to form a base.

Conjugate base A substance which can gain an H^+ ion to form an acid.

Conjugation In biology, special form of isogamy where the reproductive protoplasts of two organisms form a common tube and fuse together.

Connective tissue Animal tissue composed of cells embedded in a matrix (gel, elastic fibers, liquid, or inorganic minerals) that includes loose, dense, and fibrous connective tissues that provide strength (bone, cartilage), storage (bone, adipose), and flexibility (tendons, ligaments).

Consensus sequence A sequence of DNA, RNA, protein or carbohydrate derived from a number of similar molecules that comprises the essential features for a particular function.

Constipation A condition in which bowel movements become difficult and rare due to small, hard, or difficult-to-pass stools.

Constitutional isomerism Isomerism between structures differing in constitution and described by different line formulae, e.g. CH_3OCH_3 and CH_3CH_2OH.

Contaminant Refers to any unwanted or undesired component in a process fluid or controlled environment.

Contamination The undesired introduction of impurities of a chemical or microbiological nature, or of foreign matter, into or onto a raw material, intermediate, or active pharmaceutical ingredient (API) during production, sampling, packaging, storage or transport.

Contig Refers to group of cloned pieces of DNA representing overlapping regions of a particular chromosome.

Continuous culture system A culture system with constant environmental conditions maintained through continual condition of nutrients and removal of wastes.

Continuous fermentation A process in which sterile medium is added without interruption to the fermentation system with a balancing withdrawal of broth for product extraction.

Contraindication A condition that renders a particular type of medication as undesirable or improper for use.

Control group Refers to the group of subjects in a controlled study that receives no treatment, receives a standard treatment, or receives a placebo.

Controlled area Area of restricted access.

Controlled-release dosage forms Controlled-release dosage forms are also known as delayed-release, sustained-action, prolonged-action, sustained-release, prolonged-release, timed-release, slow-release, extended-action, and extended-release forms. They are designed to release drug substance slowly to provide prolonged action in the body.

Conventional drugs New compounds made up by chemical synthesis or fermentation, termed by the FDA as new chemical entities.

Convergent Converging together, typically of organs with their bases separate and their appices approaching each other, not touching or fused.

Convergent evolution Development of similar structures in distantly related organisms as a result of settling into similar environments and/or strategies of life (wings of birds).

Convex Having surface that curves outward.

Convulsion An abnormal, violent, and involuntary contraction or sequences of contractions of the muscles.

Coppicing Word describing the woodland management in which trees are cut back 1 m above the ground level.

Corallin soda Staining agent that stains the starch grains, lignified walls and the callus of the sieve tube.

Cordial Refers to a stimulating medicine or drink.

Coriaceous Refers to leathery texture.

Cork Refers to the suberised tissue cut off externally from the cork cambium.

Cork cambium A lateral meristem cutting off cork externally and phelloderm internally or a layer of lateral meristematic tissue between the cork and the phloem in the bark of woody plants.

Corm Refers to an enlarged solid subterranean stem, frequently rounded in shape but of no distinct characteristic shape or size in some species, filled with nutrients and composed of two or more internodes and covered externally by a few thin membranous scales or cataphyllary leaves.

Corn steep liquor It is an ingredient in the culture medium for producing penicillin and is a natural nitrogenous material that is a by-product of the corn milling industry.

Corolla The inner, usually colored or otherwise differentiated, whorl or whorls of the perianth (the petals of a flower as a whole).

Coronary arteries Arteries that supply the heart's muscle fibers with nutrients and oxygen.

Corpus callosum Refers to tightly bundled nerve fibers that connect the right and left hemispheres of the cerebrum.

Corpus luteum A structure formed from the ovulated follicle in the ovary that secretes progesterone and estrogen.

Corrosive Refers to any chemical that causes visible destruction or irreversible alterations in living tissue by chemical action at the site of contact or substance that has a corrosive or acidic substance capable of harming, burning, or eating away tissues.

Corrosive liquid Any liquid which when in contact with living tissue, will cause destruction or irreversible alteration of such tissue by chemical action.

Cortex Refers to the tissue between the phloem and the epidermis in roots and stems.

Cortical Related to the cortex.

Cortisol The primary glucocorticoid hormone that released by the adrenal cortex.

Cosmeceuticals A category of cosmetic products that produce or claim to produce therapeutic benefits.

Cotyledon The first leaf or leaves of a seed plant (seed leaves), found in the embryo of the seed which may form the first photosynthetic leaves or may remain below ground.

Coumestans A class of flavonoids derived from isoflavones, which have a coumarin structure.

Counterclockwise In plants, of the direction of twining, the stem taking an ascending counter-clockwise course when viewed from above.

Countercurrent flow Refers to an arrangement by which fish obtain oxygen from the water that flows through their gills. Water flows across the respiratory surface of the gill in one direction while blood flows in the other direction through the blood vessels on the other side of the surface.

Counterirritant An agent that causes a distracting irritation anticipated to relieve another irritation.

Coupling constant (spin-spin coupling constant) A quantitative measure for nuclear spin-spin, nuclear-electron and electron-electron coupling in magnetic resonance spectroscopy.

Covalent bonds When two atoms share at least one pair of electrons.

Cover crops Cultivation of a second type of crop primarily to improve the production system for a primary crop.

CPMP Committee for Proprietary Medicinal Products.

Crawler The active first instar of a scale insect.

Creaming Creaming is the reversible separation of a layer of emulsified particles. Because mixing or shaking may be sufficient to reconstitute the emulsion system, creaming is not necessarily unacceptable.

Cremocarp A schizocarpic fruit developed from bicarperllary syncarpous inferior ovary and is bilicular and two seeded. This fruit at maturity splits into two, one-seeded and one-chambered mericarps along the carpophore,

e.g. fruits of umbelliferae (fennel, coriander, etc.).

Crenate In leaves, of margins with small, rounded teeth or scalloped.

Cristarque cells Refers to sclereids, the lignin deposited excentrically in a U shape, that also contain a druse.

Critical A material, process step, or process condition, test requirement, or any other related parameter is considered critical when non-compliance with predetermined criteria directly influences the quality attributes of the API (active pharmaceutical ingredient) in a harmful manner.

Critical device A device that directly ensures that a GMP critical parameter is maintained within predetermined limits (e.g. terminal HEPA filter, point of use filter). A malfunction of such a device would place product quality at risk.

Critical micelle concentration (cmc) Small range of concentrations separating the limit below which virtually no micelles are detected and the limit above which virtually all additional surfactant molecules form micelles.

Critical point The combination of pressure and temperature at which the gas and liquid phases of a substance become indistinguishable.

Cross-contamination The measurable and harmful contamination of a material or product with another material or product.

Cross-pollination Refers to the pollination of one plant by another.

Cross-resistance In pest management, resistance of a pest population to a pesticide to which it has not been exposed that accompanies the development of resistance to a pesticide to which it has been exposed.

Crossing-over Term used for describing the exchange of corresponding segments of two chromatids of homologous chromosomes during meiosis that takes place by the breaking and reunion of the chromatids, and results in the independent separation of the genes.

Crown The part of a tree or shrub above the level of the lowest branch.

Crown gall A gall disease (tumourous growth) that is caused by soil borne becterium *Agrobacterium tumefaciens*.

Cruciferous Refers to stomata, anisocytic.

Crude drug Natural products that are not pure compounds (i.e. plants or parts of plants, extracts, or exudates).

Crustaceans A large taxonomic class of arthropods that includes lobsters, shrimps and crabs.

Crustaceous Brittle.

Cryogenic liquid A fluid that has a normal boiling point below-150°F (–101.1°C).

Cryoglobulins Refers to the blood proteins that stick together to form a gel when exposed to temperatures below that which is normal for a healthy human being.

Cryopreservation Ultra-low temperature storage of cells, tissues, embryos and seeds.

Cryptins Refers to peptides produced by Paneth cells in the intestines. They are toxic for some bacteria, although their mode of action is not known.

Cryptogam Exactly a plant whose sexual reproductive parts are not conspicuous.

Cryptophyte Plants with resting buds below the surface of the ground or in water.

Cryptoxanthin A carotenoid that's been associated with a decreased risk of cervical cancer.

Crystal violet Chemically hexamethyl-p-rosaniline hydrochloride, $C_{25}H_{30}N_3Cl$, an acid-base indicator that changes from green to blue as the pH passes through 1.0.

CSF Abbreviation for cerebrospinal fluid, a clear liquid contained in the spinal cord that is used in the diagnosis of some diseases.

Cucurbitacins Triterpenoids, sometimes coloured, bitter in taste.

Culm The jointed stem of grasses.

Cultivar Refers to a specially developed agricultural plant variety.

Culture Used for the growth of organisms, especially microrganisms, under clearly defined conditions which are usually artificial.

Culture medium A mixture of nutrients which is used to support the growth of a culture of microogranisms, cells, tissues, etc. It may be solid if mixed with a gelling agent (commonly agar) or liquid (absence of agar). A culture medium must have all the micro- and macronutrients that are necessary for the growth of culture and a carbohydrate source is also necessary.

Cuneate Wedge-shaped, triangular with acute angle downward.

Cuoxam Chemical that dissolves the cellulose wall.

Cupping The use of warmed glass jars to create suction on definite points of the body.

Cupule Like a small cup, cupuliform, nearly hemispherical, shaped like a cupola or dome.

Curcumins Refers to phenolic compounds, orange yellow in colour.

Cuspidate Tipped with a short, rigid point.

Cutaneous A term that refers to the skin.

Cutaneous vasculitis Skin lesions which result from inflammation and injury in the blood vessels of the skin.

Cuticle It is a continuous layer of fatty substances covering over the outer surfaces of the epidermis of plants. It contains cutin and protects against water and gases.

Cutin A waxy substance which, together with cellulose, forms the outer layer of the skin of many plants.

Cyanogenesis Production of hydrocyanic acid by hydrolysation of cyanogenic glycosides.

Cyanobacteria Refers to blue-green bacteria, unicellular or filamentous chains of cells that carry out photosynthesis.

Cyathium Type of inflorescence, consisting of a cup-like involucre bearing unisexual flowers, staminate on its inner face and pistillate from the base.

Cybotactic region That part of a solution in the surrounding area of a solute molecule in which the ordering of the solvent molecules is modified by the presence of the solute molecule. The term solvent "cosphere" of the solute has also been used.

Cybrids Cybrids or cytoplasmic hybrids are cells or plants containing nucleus of one species but cytoplasm from both the parental species.

Cycadeoids A group of gymnosperm seed plants not closely rated to, but apparently similar to, the cycads.

Cycads Group of gymnosperm seed plants which have large fern-like leaves and reproduce by cones but not flowers.

Cyclin A protein found in the dividing cells of many organisms that acts as a control during cell division.

Cyclization In chemistry, formation of a ring compound from a chain by formation of a new bond.

Cycloaddition It is a reaction in which two or more unsaturated molecules (or parts of the same molecule) combine with the formation of a cyclic adduct in which there is a net reduction of the bond multiplicity.

Cycloelimination Cycloelimination is the reverse of cycloaddition. The term also referes to "cyclo-reversion", "retro-addition", and "retrocycloaddition".

Cyclopentenoids Cyanogenic glycosides producing hydrocyanic acid, often found as cyclopentenyl fatty acids.

Cyme A cluster of flowers in which each main and secondary stem bears a single flower, the bud on the main stem blooming first, also, inflorescence in which each growing point ends in a flower.

Cymose That bears a cyme or cymes.

Cyst A general term used for a specialized microbial cell enclosed in a wall. They are formed by protozoa and a few bacteria.

Cystic fibrosis Refers to an inherited disease in which thick mucus clogs the lungs and blocks the ducts of the pancreas.

Cystisine A quinolizidine alkaloid.

Cystitis Inflammation of the bladder.

Cystolith A mass of calcium carbonate concretion, occasionally silica, formed on ingrowths of cell walls in some plants.

Cytochrome A heme protein which transfers electrons and exhibits intense absorption bands between 510 and 615 nm in the reduced form.

Cytochrome P-450 General term for a group of heme-containing mono-oxygenases. Named so because of the prominent absorption band of the Fe(II)-carbonyl complex. The heme consists of protophorphyrin IX, and the proximal ligand to iron is a cysteine sulfur.

Cytochrome-c oxidase An enzyme (ferrocytochrome-c:dioxygen oxidoreductase, cytochrome aa$_3$) and the major respiratory protein of animal and plant mitochondria, it catalyzes the oxidation of Fe(II)-cytochrome c, and the reduction of dioxygen to water.

Cytokine A protein that acts as a chemical messenger to stimulate cell migration, usually toward where the protein is released. Interleukins, lymphokines, and interferons are the most common.

Cytokinesis It is a process of cell division, as opposed to nuclear division.

Cytokinin (kinin) Growth substances which primarily stimulate cell division and the effect occurs only in association with auxin. Different proportions of auxin and cytokinin may induce different types of meristematic activity.

Cytology The branch of biology dealing with cell structure.

Cytolysis Dissolution of cells particularly by destruction of their cell membrane.

Cytopathic Damaging to cells.

Cytoplasm Refers to the part of protoplasm in a cell outside of and surrounding the nucleus.

Cytosine A pyrimidine occurring as a fundamental unit or base of nucleic acids.

Cytostatic agents Therapeutics that inhibit cell division and growth.

Cytotoxic Poisonous to cells.

Cytotaxonomy Term used to describe the number, structure and behaviour of chromosomes in taxonomic work.

D

D value The time under a stated set of exposure conditions (temperature in an autoclave) required to decrease a microbial population by a factor of 90%.

Dalton The unit of molecular weight, equal to the weight of a hydrogen atom.

Damping-off Term refers to the destruction of seedlings by one or a combination of pathogens that weaken the stem or root.

Dark-field microscopy Microscopy in which the specimen is brightly illuminated while the background is dark.

Dark reactions The sequence of light-independent reactions utilizing the energy, in the form of ATP and reducing power in the form of NADPH that are formed during the light reactions to reduce carbon dioxide.

Dating Word refers to the determination of the age of rocks, minerals and organic matter.

Daughter isotope In a nuclear equation, the compound remaining after the original isotope has undergone decay. A compound undergoing decay, e.g. alpha decay, will break into an alpha particle and a daughter isotope.

Daughter plants Vegetative progeny of plants, plants that develop along the runners produced by another plant called the mother plant.

Day neutral plants Refers to plants that flower regardless of day length.

DDD Defined daily dose.

De novo design Design of bioactive compounds by incremental construction of a ligand model within a model of the receptor or enzyme active site, the structure of which is known from X-ray or nuclear magnetic resonance (NMR) data.

Death rate The ratio between deaths and individuals in a specified population at a particular time.

Decarboxylated iridoids A kind of route II iridoid derived from epi-deoxyloganic acid via decarboxylation at the C_{11} position.

Decay Change of an element into a different element, frequently with some other particle(s) and energy emitted.

Deciduous Falling after completion of the normal function or trees that lose the leaves and have a dormancy period at least once per year.

Decoction A tea made from boiling plant material, usually the bark, rhizomes, roots or other woody parts, in water.

Decomposition The breakdown of a single entity into two or more fragments.

Decongestant Relieves congestion.

Decontamination Refers to a process that reduces contaminating substances to a defined acceptance level.

Decumbent Of stems, spreading horizontally but then growing upwards.

Decurrent That extending downward, applied usually to leaves in which the blade is apparently prolonged downward as two wings along the petiole or along the stem.

Decurved Angled downwards and curved or curled.

Defined medium Any culture medium made with components of known composition.

Definite Of a constant number.

Deflagration Refers to an exothermic reaction, such as the extremely rapid oxidation of a combustible dust or flammable vapor in air, in which the reaction progresses through the unburned material at a rate less than the velocity of sound. It can have an explosive effect.

Deflexed Bent abruptly downwards.

Deglycosylation Removal of a sugar unit (i.e. glucose) from a larger molecule called glycoside.

Dehiscence Opening and shedding contents, refers to stamens and fruits.

Dehydrogenase An oxidoreductase that catalyzes the removal of hydrogen atoms from a substrate.

Deionization Removing dissolved ions from solution by passing the solution through a bed of ion exchange resin, which consists of polymer beads that exchange hydrogen ions for cations and hydroxyl ions for anions in solution. The ionic impurities remain bound to the resins and the hydrogen and hydroxyl ions combine with each other to form water.

Delayed dormant Refers to the treatment period in fruit tree crops, beginning when buds begin to swell until the beginning of green tip development.

Deletion The loss of a chromosome segment without altering the number of chromosomes.

Delirium A mental disturbance characterized by hallucinations, confusion and disturbed speech.

Delphinidin An anthocyanin.

De minimis release The release of viable microbiological agents or eukaryotic cells that does not result in the establishment of disease in healthy people, plants, or animals.

Dementia Severe impairment of mental functioning.

Demethylation Removal of a methyl group ($:CH_3$) from a molecule.

Demineralization At times used interchangeably with deionization, refers to the removal of minerals and mineral salts using ion exchange. Water softening is a common form of demineralization.

Demulcent An oily or mucilaginous substance that soothes irritated tissue, especially mucous membranes.

Demyelination Loss of myelin, the white insulating matter covering nerve cells.

Denaturation Loss of the native structure of a macromolecule due to heat treatment, extreme pH changes, chemical treatment, etc. which is accompanied by loss of biological activity. For example, proteins may be denatured by heat, pH extremes, or addition of agents such as urea.

Denitrification The reduction of nitrates to nitrites, nitrogen monoxide (nitric oxide), dinitrogen oxide (nitrous oxide) and ultimately dinitrogen, which is catalyzed by microorganisms.

Dendritic Refers to a trichome, with branches arising along the main axis, i.e. tree-like.

Dendrochronology Refers to the process of determining the age of a tree or wood used in structures by counting the number of annual growth rings.

Dense A compact substance or a substance with a high density.

Density Mass per unit volume of a substance.

Dentifrice Substance used for cleaning teeth and gums.

Dendrochronology The process of determining the age of a tree or wood by counting the number of annual growth rings.

Deobstruent Substance that aids in the removal of obstructions, especially those lodged in organs such as stones.

Deodorant Substance that either removes, destroys, masks, or suppresses odor.

Deoxyanthocyanins Red colored flavonoids.

Deoxyribonucleic acid (DNA) A high-molecular-mass linear polymer, composed of nucleotides containing 2-deoxyribose and linked between positions 3' and 5' by phosphodiester groups. It contains the genetic information of organisms.

Depressant Substance that lessens or depresses nervous sensation, lowers a functional activity or reduces vital energy by causing the relaxation of muscles, nerves, or tissues.

Depressed Flattened as if pressed down from the top or end.

Depression A mental state of depressed mood characterized by feelings of sadness, despair and discouragement.

Depurative Tends to purify and cleanse the blood.

Depyrogenation Removal or destruction of endotoxins.

Derivative Chemicals that are made from their parent compounds are known as derivatives of the parent compound.

Dermal-epidermal junction Refers to the junction between the epidermis and dermis in the skin.

Dermatitis Refers to skin inflammation of any type or cause.

Dermatomyositis An autoimmune disease in which the skin and muscles, especially those in the shoulders and hips, are damaged with a distinctive pattern of inflammation.

Dermis The underlying, supportive layer of the skin. Collagen molecules in the dermis are responsible for structure and toughness of the skin.

Desalination Removal of dissolved salts from sea water to produce drinkable water.

Design specification A specification that defines the design of a system or system component.

Desiccant Chemical salt used to dehumidify air and to control moisture in materials contacting that air.

Desiccators Closed containers, usually made of glass or plastic, with an airtight seal used for drying materials.

Detachment The reverse of an attachment.

Detergent Cleanser.

Determinate Refers to plants, having stems and branches that stop growing at a certain point, usually after producing flowers.

Determination of shelf-life The shelf-life of a drug preparation is the amount of time that the product can be stored before it becomes unfit for use, through either chemical decomposition or physical deterioration.

Detonation Refers to an exothermic reaction characterized by the presence of a shock wave in a material that establishes and maintains the reaction. The reaction zone steps forward through the material at a rate greater than the velocity of sound.

Deuteromycetes Molds that cannot reproduce by sexual means.

Diacytic Of stomata, with two subsidiary cells surrounding the guard cells, their radial walls at right angles to the long axis of the guard cells.

Diagnosis The determination of the nature of a disease.

Diallelocytic Of stomata, with an alternating complex of three or more C-shaped subsidiary cells of graded sizes at right angles to guard cells, which is a variant of diacytic.

Dialypetalous Polypetalous.

Dialysis The separation of low-molecular weight compounds from high molecular weight components by diffusion through a semipermeable membrane.

Diaphanous Extremely thin and transparent.

Diaphoretic Substance taken internally to promote sweating.

Diaphragm A dome-shaped muscle that separates the thoracic and abdominal cavities.

Diaschistic Term used for tetrads which divide once transversely and once longitudinally, in meiosis.

Diastase An enzyme complex that breaks down starch to glucose.

Diastereoisomerism Diastereo-isomers (or diastereomers) are stereoisomers not related as mirror images and are characterised by differences in physical properties, and by some differences in chemical behaviour towards achiral as well as chiral reagents. Also referred as stereoisomerism other than enantiomerism.

Diastereomeric ratio Diastereo-meric ratio is defined by analogy with enantiomeric ratio as the ratio of the percentage of one diastereoisomer in a blend to that of the other.

Diastereomers Diastereomers are stereoisomers, which are neither mirror images nor super-imposable.

Diastereomorphism Refers to the relationship between objects analogous to that between diastereoisomeric molecular entities.

Diastole Filling of the ventricle of the heart with blood.

Diathermy Refers to deep-heat therapy that uses high-frequency electric currents to produce heat in body tissues. It is used to treat arthritis, bursitis, sinusitis and fractures.

Diatomaceous earth Siliceous geological deposits made up of diatom frustules.

Diatoms Term used for unicellular or colonial non-flagellate algae which have delicately sculptured sillica cell walls divided into two overlapping halves. Their cell walls are extremely resistant to decay and forms diatomaceous earth (kieselguhr) in lake or ocean beds.

Dichotomous Having or consisting of a pair or pairs.

Diclinous Having the stamens and the carpels in separate flowers.

Dicots One of the two main types of flowering plants which is characterized by having two cotyledons, floral organs arranged in cycles of four or five, and leaves with reticulate veins.

Dicotyledon Refers to a paraphyletic group of angiosperms with broad leaves and two cotyledons.

Dictyosomes They are also known as the Golgi apparatus. These are organelles in plant cells composed of a series of flattened membrane sacs, which sort, chemically modify, and package proteins produced on the rough endoplasmic reticulum.

Dielectric constant A measure for the effect of a medium on the potential energy of interaction between two charges and it is measured by comparing the capacity of a capacitor with and without the sample present.

Dienophile The olefin component of a Diels-Alder reaction.

Dietary supplement A product intended to supply nutrients and other healthful substances that may be lacking in a diet. Term used to apply only to vitamins, minerals, and proteins. Herbs are now classified as dietary supplements, and the definition also includes amino acids, glandulars (processed animal glands), enzymes, fish oils, and various extracts, such as flower essences. While their labels may not make any claims to cure, prevent, treat, or mitigate a disease, they can claim to help a structure or function of the body. Unlike food additives and prescription and over-the-counter drugs, dietary supplements do not require FDA approval to be sold on the market.

Differential media Culture media that differentiate between groups of microorganisms based on differences in their growth and metabolic products.

Differential staining procedures Various staining procedures that divide bacteria into separate groups based on staining properties.

Diffuse growth Refers to generalized growth, not localized at apex or base

Diffuse porous Of wood, with vessels scattered throughout the year's growth.

Diffusion The random thermal motion of particles that causes them to flow from a region of higher concentration to one of lower concentration until they are uniformly distributed.

Digestive system One of the eleven major body organ systems in animals, which converts food from the external environment into nutrient molecules that can be used and stored by the body and eliminates solid wastes. It involves five functions: movement, secretion, digestion, absorption, and elimination.

Digestives Substances that assist the stomach and intestines in normal digestion.

Digitate Palmate.

Dihydrochalcones A class of colorless flavonoids that are derived from chalcones by reduction of the alpha, beta double bond.

Dihydroflavones Flavanones.

Diluents Diluents are fillers designed to make up the required bulk of the tablet when the drug dosage amount is inadequate, Diluents may also improve cohesion, permit direct compression, or promote flow.

Dilution Lowering the concentration of a solution by adding more solvent.

Dilution factor The ratio of solvent to solute by volume.

Dimorphism Phenomenon in which an individual has an organ in two morphologically distinct forms.

Dinoflagellates Term used for describing flagellate, unicellular, marine algal members of class Dinophyceae of division Dinophyta (Pyrrophyta). They are abundant in phytoplankton and often dark-brown in colour, they have characteristically one longitudinal and one transverse groove in the cell wall and two flagella in each groove.

Dioecious Plant having unisexual flowers, the male and female flowers on different individual plants.

Dioxygenase Refers to an enzyme that catalyzes the insertion of two oxygen atoms into a substrate, both oxygens being derived from O_2.

Diploid Having twice the number of chromosomes usually occurring in a germ cell.

Dipolar bond Refers to the bond formed by coordination of two neutral moieties, the combination of which results in charge-separated structures.

Dipole-dipole forces Intermolecular forces that exist between polar molecules and active only when the molecules are close together. Their strengths of attractions increase when polarity increases.

Dipole-dipole interaction Intermolecular or intramolecular interaction between molecules or groups having a permanent electric dipole moment and the strength of the interaction depends on the distance and relative orientation of the dipoles.

Disability Lack of an ability to perform an activity in the manner that is considered normal for a human being.

Disaccharides Refers to sugars made up of two monosaccharides held together by a covalent bond, e.g. sucrose.

Discoid lupus erythematosus (DLE) Coin-shaped, scarring lupus skin lesions which occur most commonly on the scalp and face.

Discutient Substance that dissolves or causes something, such as a tumor, to disappear. Also called as discussive.

Disinfectant Destroys disease germs and noxious properties of fermentation.

Disintegrants Disintegrants are added to tablet formulations to facilitate disintegration when the tablet contacts water in the gastrointestinal tract. Disintegrants function by drawing water into the tablet, swelling, and causing the tablet to burst.

Disk Refers to a type of cultivator made up of many circular blades used for weed control and soil preparation.

Dismutase An enzyme which catalyzes a disproportionation reaction.

Dispersal mechanism Mechanism by which a propagule (seed, some other structure) of a plant is removed from the vicinity of the parent plant.

Dispersion Refers to a stable or unstable system of fine particles, evenly distributed in a medium.

Dissimilation A process, breakdown of food material to yield energy and building blocks for cellular synthesis.

Dissimilatory Refers to the conversion of food or other nutrients into products plus energy-containing compounds.

Dissociation Breaking down of a compound into its components. Also, dissociation is the separation of ions in solution when the ions are associated by interionic attraction.

Dissolved solids The amount of nonvolatile matter dissolved in a water sample, generally expressed in parts per million (PPM) by weight.

Distal Farthest away from the point of attachment or source.

Distal tubule Refers to the section of the renal tubule where tubular secretion occurs.

Distillation The process of separating water from impurities by heating until it changes into vapor and then cooling the vapor to condense it into purified water.

Distomer A distomer is the enantiomer of a chiral compound that is the less potent for a particular action.

Diterpenes C_{20} compounds made up of four isoprene units.

Dithiolthiones Refer to organosulfur compounds that are abundant in cruciferous vegetables and may aid the enzymes that fend off carcinogens and other outside invaders.

Diuretic An herb or substance that increases the secretion, flow, and expulsion of urine.

Diuretic salt Potassium acetate, KC_2H_3O.

Divergent Separated from one another, having tips further apart than the bases.

Divergent evolution Refers to the divergence of a single interbreeding population or species into two or more descendant species.

DMF Drug master file.

DMSO Dimethyl sulfoxide.

DNase (deoxyribonuclease) Refers to an enzyme that degrades DNA.

DNA hybridization The formation of hybrid DNA molecules, which contain a strand of DNA from two different species. The number of complementary sequences in common in the two strands is an indication of the degree of relatedness of the species.

DNA ligase In recombinant DNA technology, an enzyme, which seals together two DNA fragments from different sources to form a recombinant DNA molecule.

DNA polymerase In DNA replication, the enzyme, which links the complementary nucleotides together to form the newly synthesized strand.

DNA replication Using the existing DNA as a template, synthesis of new DNA strands. It occurs in the cell nucleus in humans and other eukaryotes.

DNA sequence The relative order of base pairs, whether in a fragment of DNA, a gene, a chromosome, or an entire genome.

DNA vector Refers to a DNA vehicle for transferring generic information from one cell to another.

DNA vaccine A vaccine that contains DNA that encodes antigenic proteins. It is injected directly into the muscle and the DNA is taken up by the muscle cells and encoded protein antigens are synthesized. This produces both humoral and cell-mediated responses.

Docking studies Docking studies are molecular modeling studies planning at finding a proper fit between a ligand and its binding site.

Domain An independently folded unit within a protein, frequently joined by a flexible segment of the polypeptide chain.

Dominant allele Refers to a gene which is expressed, regardless of whether its counterpart allele on the other chromosome is dominant or recessive. Single mutated dominant allele, even though its corresponding allele is normal produces autosomal dominant disorders.

Dopamine Refers to a compound found in the nervous and peripheral tissues of the body, also the immediate precursor of noradrenaline with the empirical formula $C_8H_{11}NO_2$.

Dormant To become inactive during winter or cold weather.

Dorsal Pertains to the back, the surface turned away from the axis.

Dorsifixed Attached at or by the back.

Dorsiventral Of bifacial structures, especially leaves, having tissues derived from the adaxial and abaxial surfaces of the leaf primordium, palisade cells below both the upper and lower epidermis.

Dosage form Refers to the form in which the drug is delivered to the patient. This could be parenteral, topical, tablet, oral, suppository, inhalation, transdermal, etc.

Dose A quantity to be administered at one time.

Dose response relationship In general, the larger the drug dose, the higher the drug concentration as its site of action and the greater the effect of the drug, up to a maximum effect. Higher drug concentration (or doses) will not produce an effect greater than the maximum effect.

Double bond When an atom is bonded to another atom by two sets of electron pairs, it refers to double bond.

Double fertilization A feature of angiosperms in which a pollen tube carries two sperm cells to the female gametophyte in the ovule. One sperm cell fuses with the egg cell and gives rise to a diploid embryo and the other sperm cell fuses with the two polar cells to form a triploid cell that develops into the endosperm.

Double prodrug (or pro-prodrug)
A double prodrug is a biologically inactive molecule that is transformed *in vivo* in two steps (enzy-

matically and/or chemically) to the active species.

Double-blind study A double-blind study is a clinical study of potential and marketed drugs, where neither the investigators nor the subjects know which subjects will be treated with the active principle and which ones will receive a placebo.

Dough stage Refers to a stage in grain development when the grain turns from a liquid to a soft doughy consistency before hardening.

Downy Covered with short, fine hairs.

Dragendroff's reagent Reagent for the detection of alkaloids.

Drift The aerial dispersal of a substance such as a pesticide beyond the intended application area.

Dropsy Refers to a disease characterized by accumulation of fluid in connective tissues and serous cavities in the body.

Drug product Refers to a finished dosage form, e.g. tablet, capsule, suspension, etc. which contains one or more APIs (active pharmaceutical ingredients) generally, but not necessarily, in association with inactive ingredients.

Drug disposition Drug disposition refers to all processes involved in the absorption, distribution metabolism and excretion of drugs in a living organism.

Drug latentiation Drug latentiation is the chemical modification of a biologically active compound to form a new compound that *in vivo* will liberate the parent compound. The term is synonymous with prodrug design.

Drug targeting Drug targeting is a strategy aiming at the delivery of a compound to a particular tissue of the body.

Drugs Refers to articles intended for use in diagnosis, cure, mitigation, treatment, or prevention of disease in man or other animals and articles (other than food) intended to affect the structure or any function of the body of man or other animals.

Drupe Refers to a succulent fruit having the seed(s) enclosed by a stony endocarp.

Dry air Refers to the air from which all water vapor and contaminants have been removed. Its composition by volume is: 1. Nitrogen 78.08%; 2. Oxygen 20.95%; 3. Argon 0.93%; 4. Carbon dioxide 0.03%; 5. Other gases 0.00003%.

Dry heat sterilization Refers to sterilization utilizing a heating oven or continuous tunnel (gas or electric heated), as opposed to steam sterilization in an autoclave, usually used for glassware and metal parts. In depyrogenation temperatures of 250°C result in sterilization and the inactivation of endotoxin present on the equipment.

Dry skin Dull, scaly skin which results from loss of water from the skin.

Dual action drug A dual action drug is a compound that combines two desired different pharmacological actions at a similarly efficacious dose.

Duodenum The upper part of the small intestine.

Duplication An extra copy of a chromosome part without altering the number of chromosomes.

Durable medical equipment (DME) An item which can withstand repeated use, is primarily used to serve a medical purpose, is generally not useful to you in the absence of illness or injury and is appropriate for use in the home.

Duramen Refers to heartwood.

Dwarfing An inhibition of normal growth characterized in plants by smaller than normal leaves and stems.

Dysentery General term for a group of diseases characterized by swelling of the mucous membrane in the large intestine with symptoms like nausea, diarrhea, ulcers, blood and mucous in stool.

Dysesthesia Abnormal sensations on the skin which include burning, prickling, numbness, or pain.

Dysoxlin Refers to a limonoid.

Dysphagia Difficulty in swallowing.

Dysphoria Refers to a feeling of unpleasantness or discomfort.

Dysploid Chromosome numbers which differ between species and do not show any regular pattern.

Dystrophin Protein making up only 0.002% of all protein in skeletal muscle but which appears vital for proper functioning of the muscle. Sufferers of muscular dystrophy appear to lack dystrophin.

Dystropic rearrangement Refers to an uncatalyzed process in which two sigma bonds simultaneously migrate intramolecularly.

E

E. coli (Escherichia coli) A fast growing, gram-negative bacteria commonly found in the body with a simple structure.

Ear candling (ear coning) Involves placing the narrow end of a specially designed hollow candle at the entry of the ear canal, while the opposite end is lit. Mainly used for relieving wax build up and related hearing problems, ear candling is also used for ear infections and sinus infections.

Early wood The wood, strictly speaking xylem, formed early in the growing period, characteristically relatively low in density, pale in colour, and with large xylem elements.

Earth A metal oxide.

Eccrine glands Sweat glands, which are linked to the sympathetic nervous system and are widely distributed over the body surface.

Eclipsed Two atoms or groups attached to neighboring atoms are said to be eclipsed if the torsion angle between the three bonds is zero.

Ecology Branch of science concerned with the interrelationships of organisms and their environments esp. as manifested by natural cycles and rhythms, community development and structure, interaction between different kinds of organisms, geographic distributions and population alteration.

Economic threshold Refers to a level of pest population or damage at which the cost of control action equals the crop value gained from control action.

Ecotype Ecotypes are examples of the same species which are found in different habitats and have evolved specific adaptations to their differing environments.

Ecovar Selections of native plant species usually collected from a large geographic area of genetic diversity that are developed by phenotypic selections for specific traits. They have somewhat greater genetic diversity than many cultivars.

Ectoparasite Refers to a parasite that lives on the outside of its host.

Ectophloic Refers to a variant of a siphonostele in which there is phloem only outside the xylem.

Eczema A chronic, non-contagious inflammation of the skin characterized by itching and the presence of skin vesicles which discharge fluid.

EDQM European Directorate for the Quality of Medicines of the Council of Europe.

Edge failure A control limit value that, if exceeded, may result in adverse effect on state of control and/or fitness for use of the product.

Effective molarity (effective concentration) The ratio of the first-order rate constant of an intramolecular reaction involving two functional groups within the same molecular entity to the second-order rate constant of an analogous intermolecular elementary reaction. This ratio has the dimension of concentration and this term can also apply to an equilibrium constant.

Effervescent tablets Effervescent tablets are prepared by compressing granular effervescent salts or other materials (e.g. citric acid, tartaric acid, sodium bicarbonate) that release carbon dioxide gas when they come into contact with water. Commercial alkalinizing analgesic tablets are often made to effervesce to encourage rapid dissolution and absorption.

Efficacy The ability of a substance to produce the desired effect.

Effluent The output or release from a process, such as a waste water treatment process.

Effusion Refers to the movement of gas molecules through a small opening.

EGA European Generic Medicines Association.

EHFG European Health Forum Gastein.

Elaters Structures of various origins either associated with individual pollen grains, or mixed among them that by their movements as they dry out cause the pollen to be dispersed.

Elastin An albuminoid, or scleroprotein that is present especially in yellow elastic fibrous tissue.

Elastomer Long chain co-polymers or terpolymers (two or three different monomers in one chain) which contain adequate crosslinks among individual chains.

Electrochemical cell Gives an electric current with a steady voltage because of an electron transfer reaction.

Electrocyclic reaction A molecular rearrangement that involves the formation of a sigma bond between the termini of a fully conjugated linear pi-electron system (or a linear fragment of a pi-electron system) and a decrease by one in the number of pi bonds, or the reverse of that process.

Electrode potential Electrode potential of an electrode is defined as the electromotive force (emf) of a cell in which the electrode on the left is a standard hydrogen electrode and the electrode on the right is the electrode in question.

Electrodes Device that moves electrons into or out of a solution by conduction.

Electrodialysis (ED) A membrane separation method used for the separation of charged molecules from a solution by application of a direct current in which the membranes contain ion-exchange groups and have a fixed electrical charge. This is an effective method in the concentration of electrolytes and proteins.

Electrofuge A leaving group which does not carry away the bonding electron pair, e.g. in the nitration of benzene by NO_2^+, H^+ is the electrofuge.

Electrolysis Using electrical energy, changing the chemical structure of a compound.

Electrolyte A chemical compound that when dissolved or ionized in water allows it to conduct electric current. Also, electrolytes are substances that do form ions in solution. Examples are sodium chloride, hydrochloric acid, and atropine.

Electromagnetic spectrum Complete range of wavelengths that light can have, which include infrared, ultraviolet, and all other types of electromagnetic radiation, as well as visible light.

Electron One of the parts of the atom, which have a negative charge or indivisible particle with a charge of -1.

Electron acceptor A substance to which an electron may be transferred.

Electron affinity The energy released when an additional electron, without excess energy, attaches itself to a molecular entity.

Electron attachment The transfer of an electron to a molecular entity, resulting in a molecular entity of increased negative charge.

Electron detachment Refers to the reverse of an electron attachment.

Electron donor A molecular entity which can transfer an electron to another molecular entity, or to the corresponding chemical species.

Electron geometry Refers to the structure of a compound based on the arrangement of its electrons.

Electron microscopy (EM) A technique for visualizing material which uses beams of electrons instead of light rays and that permits greater magnification than is possible with an optical microscope.

Electron paramagnetic resonance (EPR) spectroscopy Refers to the form of spectroscopy concerned with microwave-induced transitions between magnetic energy levels of electrons having a net spin and orbital angular momentum. The spectrum is normally obtained by magnetic field scanning and is also known as electron spin resonance (ESR) spectroscopy or electron magnetic resonance (EMR) spectroscopy.

Electron spin-echo (ESE) spectroscopy A pulsed method in electron paramagnetic resonance, in some ways analogous to pulsed methods in NMR. It can be used for measurements of electron spin relaxation times as they are influenced by neighbouring paramagnets or molecular motion and also to measure anisotropic nuclear hyperfine couplings.

Electron transfer Transfer of an electron from one molecular entity to another, or between two localized sites in the same molecular entity.

Electron transfer protein A protein, often containing a metal ion, which oxidizes and reduces other molecules by means of electron transfer.

Electron-deficient bond A single bond between adjacent atoms which is formed by less than two electrons.

Electronegativity Measuring the power of an atom or a group of atoms to attract electrons from other parts of the same molecular entity.

Electroneutrality principle The principle states the fact that all pure substances carry a net charge of zero.

Electron-nuclear double resonance (ENDOR) A magnetic resonance spectroscopic method for the determination of hyperfine interactions between electrons and nuclear spins.

Electrophile (electrophilic) An electrophile or electrophilic reagent is a reagent which forms a bond to its reaction partner, the nucleophile by accepting both bonding electrons from that reaction partner.

Electrophoresis Refers to the migration of electrically charged proteins, colloids, molecules, or other particles when dissolved or suspended in an electrolyte through which an electric current is passed. Also it is a technique that separates substances through differences in their migration rate in an electrical field due to variations in the number and kinds of charged groups they have.

Electropolishing (chemical machining) (reverse plating) It is an electrochemical process far superior to any available mechanical process for the removal of minute surface imperfections in stainless steel. It levels and brightens the material surface by anodic dissolution in an electrolyte flowing solution with an forced electrical current.

Electroporation The application of an electric field to create temporary pores in the plasma membrane in order to insert foreign materials into the cell and transform it.

Electrostatic attraction The attraction between atoms of opposite charge which holds the atoms together in ionic bonds.

Electrostatic fluidized bed A container holding powder coating material that is aerated from below so as to form an air-supported expanded cloud of such material which is electrically charged with a charge opposite to the charge of the object to be coated. Such object is transported through the container immediately above the charged and aerated materials to be coated.

Electrostatic forces Refers to the forces between charged objects.

Element Substance consisting of only one type of atom.

Elementary reaction A reaction for which no reaction intermediates have been detected or need to be postulated in order to describe the chemical reaction on a molecular scale. This reaction is assumed to occur in a single step and to pass through a single transition state.

ELISA (enzyme linked immunosorbent assay) A test to measure the concentration of antigens or antibodies.

Ellagic acid Refers to a lactone, a hydroxy acid formed by the hydrolysis of some tannins, for the combined state.

Ellagitannins Hydrolyzable tannins, ester involving dimers of gallic acid.

Elliptic Of shape, an outline that is oval, narrowed to rounded at the ends and widest at about the middle. Ellipsoid, a solid with an elliptical outline.

Elixirs Elixirs are traditionally peroral solutions that contain alcohol as a consolvent.

Elute To separate one solute from another by washing. Elution may comprise the removal by means of a suitable solvent of one material (absorbed material) from another (adsorbent) that is insoluble in that solvent.

Emarginate Refers to leaves, sepals, or petals, and other structures that are notched at the apex.

Embriology The study of the early stages in the development of an organism.

Embryo culture *In vitro* culture of isolated mature or immature embryos.

Embryo sac It is a part of the ovule, a large, multi-nucleate structure, the whole making up the female gametophyte, in which an embryo begins to develop.

Embryo A young plant contained within a seed.

EMEA The European Medicines Agency that is responsible for evaluating medicinal products and providing advice on research and development programmes and maintaining various databases available to healthcare professionals and the public.

Emenagogue An herb or substance that promotes and regulates menstrual flow.

Emerge To rise out of a fluid or other covering.

Emersed Rising above the surface of water in which the plant is rooted.

Emetic A substance that induces vomiting.

Emollient Another name for moisturizers that is used externally to soften and soothe irritated skin, inflamed tissue, or mucous membranes.

Empirical formula Formula showing the simplist ratio of elements in a compound.

EMR Acronym for electron magnetic resonance.

Emulsifying agent Any compound that lowers the interfacial tension and forms a film at the interface can potentially function as an emulsifying agent.

Emulsion It is a mixture of two immiscible substances, one substance (the dispersed phase) is dispersed in the other (the continuous phase). An emulsion is a heterogeneous system that consists of at least one immiscible liquid that is intimately dispersed in another in the form of droplets. The droplet diameter usually exceeds 0.1 μm.

Emulsion bases Emulsion bases may be w/o emulsions, which are water-insoluble and are not washable in water. These emulsions can absorb water because of their aqueous internal phase. Emulsion bases may also be o/w emulsions, which are water-insoluble, but washable in hey can absorb water in their aqueous external phase.

Enantiomers Enantiomers are optical isomers that are mirror images of one another. Enantiomers have identical physical and chemical properties except that one rotates the plane of polarized light in a clockwise direction (dextrorotatory, designated Q or +) and the other in a counterclockwise direction (levorotatory, designated L or -).

Enantiomerically pure A sample all of whose molecules have the same chirality sense.

Enantiomerisation The interconversion of enantiomers.

Enantiomerism The isomerism of enantiomers.

Enantiomorph One of a pair of chiral objects or models which are non-superposable mirror images of each other. The adjective enantiomorphic is also applied to mirror-image related groups within a molecular entity.

Enantiotopic Constitutionally identical atoms or groups in molecules that are related by symmetry elements of the second kind only.

Endangered species A species that is facing imminent extirpation or extinction.

Endarch Of a procambial strand in that the first differentiated elements are in the inside, i.e. towards the centre of the stem.

Endemic A disease present in a community or among a group of people or used to describe a disease prevailing continually in a region.

Endemic species A native species whose distribution is comparatively restricted to a certain region.

Endocarp The innermost histologically different layer of the fruit wall or pericarp, in a drupe.

Endocrine glands The glands which secrete their products (hormones) into the blood that then carries them to their specific target organs. They are the pituitary, thyroids, adrenals, pancreas, ovaries (in females), and testes (in males).

Endocrine hormones The products secreted by the endocrine glands.

Endocrine system One of eleven major body organ systems in animals and it is a system of glands that works with the nervous system in controlling the activity of internal organs, especially the kidneys, and in coordinating the long-range response to external stimuli.

Endocytic Living inside a cell.

Endocytosis Refers to the process in which a cell takes up solutes or particles by enclosing them in vesicles pinched off from its plasma membrane.

Endodermis Refers to the innermost layer of the cortex, consisting of a single layer of cells without intercellular spaces.

Endogenous Biochemicals that are made by and within the human body are called endogenous, as opposed to exogenous, those which come from outside.

Endometrium The inner lining of the uterus.

Endonuclease An enzyme which cleaves its nucleic acid substrate at internal sites (other than the terminal bonds) in the nucleotide sequence.

Endoparasite A parasite which lives inside its host.

Endoplasmic reticulum A network of membranous tubules in the cytoplasm of a cell that is involved in the production of phospholipids, proteins, and for other functions.

ENDOR Acronym for electron-nuclear double resonance.

Endorphins Endogenous opiates having morphine-like effects consisting of small polypeptides such as enkephalin and leu-enkephalin and longer polypeptides such as alpha-, beta-, and gamma-endorphins. They bind to opiate receptors in the brain.

Endoskeleton An internal supporting skeleton with muscles on the outside; in vertebrates, consists of the skull, spinal column, ribs, and appendages.

Endosperm Nutritive tissue in an angiosperm seed, usually triploid, sometimes diploid or polyploid, and formed after fertilisation by the fusion of one gamete with the polar nucleus.

Endoplasm Refers to the central portion of the cytoplasm in a protozoan.

Endoplasmic reticulum A system of membranous tubules and flattened sacs (cisternae) in the cytoplasmic matrix of eucaryotic cells.

Endospore A highly heat and chemical resistant dormant inclusion (spore) taking place within the substance of certain genera of bacteria, mainly Bacillus and Clostridium.

Endosymbiosis Theory, which attempts to explain the origin of the DNA-containing mitochondria and chloroplasts in early eukaryotes by the engulfing of various types of bacteria, which were not digested but became permanent additions to the ancestral eukaryote.

Endothelial cells A layer of flat cells which line the tumor blood vessel structure.

Endothermic Reaction which absorbs heat from its surroundings as the reaction proceeds.

Endotoxin A poisonous complex molecule (lipopolysaccharide) which forms an integral part of the bacterial (gram-negative bacteria) cell wall and is only released when the integrity of the wall is disturbed. Also certain organisms may release endotoxins (e.g. *E. coli*) during biosynthesis of a recombinant DNA product, thus necessitating purification steps to ensure their removal.

Ene reaction The addition of a compound with a double bond having an allylic hydrogen, the "ene", to a compound with a multiple bond, the "enophile", with transfer of the allylic hydrogen and a concomitant reorganization of the bonding is known as Ene reaction.

Energy Ability to do work.

Energy of activation The minimum amount of energy required for a given reaction to occur and it varies from reaction to reaction.

Ensiform Of shape, having sharp edges and tapering to a slender point; having a shape suggesting a sword.

Ent A prefix used to specify the enantiomer for natural products and related molecules where the trivial name only refers to one enantiomers. For example, *Ent*-kaurene is the enantiomer of kaurene.

Entatic state A state of an atom or group which due to its binding to a protein, has its geometric or electronic condition adapted for function.

Enteric-coated Enteric-coated tablets are coated and remain intact in the stomach, but yield their ingredients in the intestines. Enteric-coated tablets are a form of delayed-action tablet. However, not all delayed action tablets are enteric or are intended to produce an enteric effect.

Enterobactin A siderophore found in enteric bacteria such as *Escherichia coli*, also called as enterochelin.

Enterotoxin A toxin specifically affecting the cells of the intestinal mucosa, causing vomiting and diarrhea.

Enthalpy Change in heat.

Entropy Measure of the disorder of a system.

Enzyme Any of numerous proteins or conjugated proteins which are produced by living organisms and functioning as complex biochemical catalysts. They also function as regulators making sure the organism does not produce too much or too little of any chemical substance. Even though all enzymes are proteins, many contain additional nonprotein components essential for catalytic activity and such enzymes are termed haloenzymes. The protein part of this enzyme is termed an apoenzyme and the non-amino acid part is termed a coenzyme.

Enzyme induction It is the process whereby an enzyme is synthesized in reply to a specific inducer molecule. The inducer molecule joins with a repressor and thereby prevents the blocking of an operator by the repressor leading to the translation of the gene for the enzyme.

Enzyme-linked immunosorbent assay A method used for detecting and quantifying specific antibodies and antigens.

Enzyme repression It is the mode by which the synthesis of an enzyme is prevented by repressor molecules.

Enzyme therapy A form of therapy that uses supplements of plant and animal enzymes to improve digestive function and other conditions.

Eophyll Refers to the first leaf or leaves produced by the seedling.

Eosinophil A polymorphonuclear leukocyte which has a two-lobed nucleus and cytoplasmic granules that stain yellow-red.

Ephedrine A protoalkaloid.

Epicotyl Refers to the part of an embryo or seedling above the attachment point of the cotyledon(s).

Epicuticular wax Wax of variable composition and morphology found on the outer surfaces of the above ground parts of plants.

Epidemic A disease attacking many people in a community simultaneously and it is distinguished from endemic, since the disease is not continuously present but has been introduced from outside.

Epidermis The outer cellular layer of the skin which produces the stratum corneum or a cellophane-type membrane that separates the skin from its environment.

Epididymis A long, convoluted duct on the testis in which sperm are stored.

Epigynous Growing upon the top of the ovary or seeming to do so, as petals, sepals, and stamens.

Epilepsy A disease of the nervous system that is characterized by convulsions, seizures, and unconsciousness.

Epilithic Living on rock or stone.

Epimer A diastereoisomer which has the opposite configuration at only one of two or more tetrahedral stereogenic centres present in the respective molecular entity, or, epimers are a special type of diastereomers because all epimers are also diastereomers; however, the opposite is not true. Epimers are compounds that are structurally identical in all respects except for the stereochemistry about one chiral center.

Epimerisation Interconversion of epimers.

Epinasty Describing the growth response of a plant part where the upper side grows faster than the lower side so that the part curves downwards.

Epinephrine A hormone produced by the adrenal medulla and secreted under stress, also contributes to the fight response.

Epipetalous Having stamens inserted on petals.

Epiphyte A plant that grows upon another plant. It does not eat the plant on which it grows, but just uses the plant for structural support, or as a way to get off the ground and into the canopy environment.

Epispastic Refers to the substances locally applied to the skin.

Epistasis The masking of the effects of one gene by the action of another.

Epistomatic Of leaves in which stomata are borne on the upper or adaxial side only.

Epithelial tissue Cells in animals, which are closely packed in either single or multiple layers, and which cover both internal and external surfaces of the animal body.

Epithelium A compact layer of cells, frequently secretory, lining a cavity or covering a surface.

Epizoic Living on an animal.

EPO (Erythropoietin) A glycoprotein hormone which stimulates the production of red blood cells and is a commercialized product of recombinant DNA technology.

Epoxy These materials are based on the reactive oxirane group that are characterized by the attachment of one oxygen atom to two different adjacent carbon atoms.

Epsom salts Refers to magnesium sulfate, $MgSO_4 \cdot 7H_2O$.

Equilibrium constant Refers to the value which expresses how far the reaction proceeds before reaching equilibrium. A small number means that the equilibrium is towards the reactants side while a large number means that the equilibrium is towards the products side.

Equilibrium expressions The expression that gives the ratio between the products and reactants. The equilibrium expression is equivalent to the concentration of each product raised to its coefficient in a balanced chemical equation and multiplied together, divided by the concentration of the product of reactants to the power of their coefficients.

Equilibrium When the reactants and products are in a constant ratio it is said to be in equilibrium. Also, the forward reaction and the reverse reactions occur at the same rate when a system is in equilibrium.

Equivelence point Happens when the moles of acid equal the moles of base in a solution.

Erect Held at right angles to the surface.

Erectile dysfunction Impotence or the incapability to develop/maintain an erection.

Ergastic substances Refers to the metabolic products of the protoplast such as starch grains, calcium oxalate crystals, fat globules, fluids, etc., which are found in various parts of the cell, including the cell wall.

Ergotism The disease or toxic condition caused by eating grain infected with ergot. It is frequently accompanied by gangrene, psychotic delusions, nervous spasms, abortion, and convulsions in humans and in animals.

Ericoid A xeromorphic leaf, quite small, narrow, and with recurved margins.

Erose Having small irregular notches in the margin, as if chewed.

Errhine Refers to herbs applied to the mucus membranes of the nose to increase nasal secretion.

Erythema or erythematous Red skin that is usually the result of inflammation.

Erythrocyte Erythrocytes also known as red blood cell, are biconcave discs that are manufactured in the bone marrow, consisting largely of hemoglobin and carrying nearly all the oxygen contained in the blood.

Erythrocyte sedimentation rate (sed rate) A laboratory test which measures the rate at which red blood cells settle in a test tube. When inflammation is present somewhere in the body, the results of this test are abnormally elevated.

Esculent Edible or fit for eating.

Esculetin Refers to a coumarin.

ESEEM Acronym for electron spin-echo envelope modulation.

ESR Acronym for electron spin resonance.

Essential amino acids Refers to the amino acids which cannot be synthesized by human and other vertebrates and must be obtained from the diet.

Essential fatty acids Refers to the group of polyunsaturated fatty acids of plants that are required in the human diet.

Essential oil Also called volatile oil (ethereal oils), any of a class of volatile oils which impart the characteristic odors of plants; used especially in perfumes, food flavorings and aromatherapy. They are made up of various kinds of terpenes, including diterpenes, sesquiterpenes, etc.

Esters Esters have a general formula of R – COOR.

Ethers Ethers have a general formula of R – O – R, with an oxygen atom bonded to two carbon atoms.

Ethical pharmaceutical Refers to a controlled substance for the diagnosis or treatment of disease.

Ethnobotany The investigation of human interactions with plants.

Ethylene A gaseous plant hormone which stimulates fruit ripening and the dropping of leaves.

Etiology The cause of disease.

Etiologic agent A disease-causing organism or toxin.

Euanthium A structure representing a single, simple flower.

Eukaryote An organism which carries its genetic material physically constrained within a nuclear membrane, separate from the cytoplasm. All animal and plant cells except bacteria, viruses, and bluegreen algae are eukaryotic and they are five to ten times larger than prokaryotes in diameter.

Euphoria A state of unrealistic happiness, joyfulness, and optimism.

Eutectic Pertaining to, or formed at the lowest possible temperature of solidification for any mixture of specified constituents.

Eutomer The eutomer is the enantiomer of a chiral compound which is the more potent for a particular action.

Eutrophic Gradual increase in nutrients in a body of water (human activities may greatly accelerate the process of eutrophication).

Eutrophication Refers to the process of becoming eutrophic.

Evaporation The part of the hydrologic cycle in which liquid water is converted to vapor and enters the atmosphere.

Evaporator An apparatus used in the process of distillation to heat a liquid and create a phase change from the liquid to the vapor state.

Evapotranspiration Refers to the loss of soil moisture due to evaporation from the soil surface and transpiration by plants.

Even-pinnate Of compound leaves having an even number of leaflets, this is easily determined because there is a pair terminally.

Evergreen Bearing green leaves throughout the year.

Exacerbation A period of time when symptoms worsen and these periods may come and go without warning and may last a few days or weeks at a time.

Exalbuminous With no endosperm.

Exanthematous Refers to any eruptive disease or fever.

Exarch Of a procambial strand in that the first differentiated elements are towards the outside.

Excentric To one side, off centre.

Excipient They are inert substance added in a prescription drug compound as a diluent or vehicle or to give form or consistency when the remedy is given in a pill form.

Excited state Refers to the state of a system with energy higher than that of the ground state. This term is frequently used to characterize a molecule in one of its electronically excited states, but can also refer to vibrational and/or rotational excitation in the electronic ground state.

Excrescence A normal outgrowth.

Excretion The process of removing the waste products of cellular metabolism from the body.

Excretory system One of the eleven major body systems in animals. It controls the volume and molecular and ionic constitution of internal body fluids and eliminates metabolic waste products from the internal environment.

Excurrent Projecting beyond the tip, the same as the midrib of a leaf or bract.

Exfoliate Refers to peeling off in thin layers, shreds, or plates, as the bark of a few trees.

Exhilarant An herb or substance that excites or elevates the psychic function, or produces an abnormal sense of euphoria, energy, and buoyancy.

Exine Outer covering of pollen grains, frequently containing sporopollenin, an acid-resistant polysaccharide that allows pollen grains to become fossils.

Exocarp Refers to the outer layer of the wall of a matured ovary.

Exoenzymes Refers to those enzymes that are secreted by cells.

Exogenous That originates externally.

Exogenous DNA Refers to DNA originating outside an organism.

Exon Refers to the protein coding DNA sequence of an eukaryotic gene.

Exonuclease An enzyme which cleaves nucleotides in sequence from free ends of a linear nucleic acid substrate.

Exosporic Growth of the gametophytic generation after germination of a spore which takes place at least in part outside the spore wall.

Exostomal Refers to the area where the micropyle of an ovule is formed from the outer integument alone.

Exothecium The epidermis of an anther sac with characteristically thickened walls and involved in its dehiscence, frequently only when this is poricidal.

Exothermic Reaction that releases off heat to the environment.

Exotic organism Refers to a biological agent where either the matching disease does not exist in a given country or geographical area, or where the disease is the issue of prophylactic measures or an elimination program undertaken in the given country or geographical area.

Exotoxins These are proteins produced by bacteria which are able to diffuse into a medium through the bacterial cell membrane and cell wall. They are usually more potent and specific in their actions than endotoxins.

Expansigenous Refers to cavities in plants, formed by cells expanding differentially by cell division and extension of walls lining the enlarging spaces.

Expectorant An herb or substance that promotes the discharge of mucus and phlegm from the lungs and throat by means of spitting and expectoration.

Expiration date The date placed on the container/labels of an active pharmaceutical ingredient (API) designating the time during which the API is expected to remain within established shelf life specifications if stored under defined conditions, and after which it should not be used.

Explant Refers to an excised piece or part of a plant used to initiate a tissue culture.

Explosive A chemical which causes a sudden, almost immediate release of pressure, gas and heat when subjected to sudden shock, pressure, or high temperatures, or a material or chemical, other than a blasting agent, which is commonly used or intended for the purpose of producing an explosive effect.

Exponential rate An extremely rapid increase, e.g., in the rate of population growth.

Exposed or open process The process that is exposed to the room environment.

Express To translate the genetic information which is stored in the DNA into protein.

Expression system A host organism combined with a genetic vector, plasmid, which is loaded with a gene of interest. The expression system provides the genetic context in which a gene will function in the cell, specifically, the gene will be expressed as a protein.

Expressive therapies Using the arts (art therapy, dance therapy, drama therapy, music therapy, poetry, and psychodrama) to promote physical and mental health and personal growth.

Exsert To protrude.

Exstipulate With no stipules.

Extirpated species Native species which no longer exist in the wild in any part of their original distribution area, though they may exist somewhere else.

Extract A preparation obtained from soaking an herb, plant part, or substance in an appropriate solvent, usually alcohol, water, or glycerine, then removing the solid parts by straining, evaporating some or all of the solvent, and adjusting the result to prescribed standards of concentration.

Extractables Undesirable foreign substances which are leached or dissolved by water or process streams from the materials of construction used in filters, storage vessels, distribution piping, and other wetted surfaces.

Extrafloral nectary A nectary located outside the flower.

Extrinsic factor An environmental factor such as temperature, rainfall, etc.

Eye (plant) A collection of several buds on the surface of a tuber, one of which will sprout and form a new stem in favorable conditions.

F-430 A component of the enzyme methyl-coenzyme M reductase, which is involved in the formation of methane in methanogenic bacteria. Also it has a tetrapyrrole structure containing nickel and the highly reduced macrocyclic structure, related to porphyrins and corrins, is termed a corphin.

Facilitated diffusion Diffusion across the plasma membrane which is aided by a carrier.

Factor VIII (hemophilia factor) Also known as antihemophilic factor (AHF) in the clotting of blood, factor VIII is a labile protein of the blood-clotting system which assists in the conversion of factor IX into plasma factor X. Deficiency of this factor is associated with classic hemophilia A, a hereditary, sex-linked, hemorrhagic tendency which occurs almost exclusively in men, characterized by prolonged clotting time, less thromboplastin is formed and the conversion of prothrombin is diminished. Factor IX (hemophilia factor): Part in the clotting of blood (Christmas factor). Deficiency of this factor causes hemophilia B or Christmas disease which resembles hemophilia A, and is an inherited defect that leads to a severe hemorrhagic disorder. It is required for the formation of intrinsic blood thromboplastin and affects the amount formed.

Facultative Exhibiting some capability or function under some environmental conditions but not under others.

Falcarinone Refers to a type of polyacetylene.

Falcate Curved similar to a sickle.

Fallow Cultivated land which is allowed to lie dormant, with no crops growing on it, during a growing season.

Family A group of one to many genera which is guessed to be monophyletic and morphologically separable from other such groups. It is a major rank in the taxonomic hierarchy between genus and order and with the termination-aceae.

Farinaceous Containing starch grains, mealy, that resembles flour.

Fascicle Refers to a small bundle or bunch, as of fibers, leaves, etc.

Fast-atom bombardment (FAB) mass spectroscopy A method in that ions are produced in a mass spectrometer from nonvolatile or thermally fragile organic molecules by bombarding the compound in the condensed phase with energy-rich neutral particles.

Fastigiate Refers to branches close to stem and erect.

Fatigue Tiredness or exhaustion.

Fats Triglycerides that are solid at room temperature.

Fatty acids Straight chain monocarboxylic acids, either saturated, with no double bonds, or unsaturated, with one or more double bonds.

Fauna Term refers collectively to all animals in an area.

FDA United States Food and Drug Administration.

Febrifuge An agent that reduces fever (also called an antipyretic).

Feces Refers to semisolid material containing undigested foods, bacteria, bilirubin, and water, which is produced in the large intestine and eliminated from the body.

Fed-Batch fermentation This is the most common operating mode for rDNA fermentation. After an initial partial charge of media to the fermenter and seed transfer, sterile media is added at measured rates during the balance of the fermentation cycle. In this case, cell mass and broth are withdrawn only at the end of the cycle.

Feeder roots Refer to the youngest roots with root hairs and are important in absorption of water and minerals.

Feedwater Refers to the water entering a treatment process.

Fehling's solution Solution used for the detection of reducing sugars.

Femur Refers to the upper leg bone.

Fen Low land covered wholly or partially with water but producing sedge, coarse grasses, or other aquatic plants. Also refers to boggy land or a moor or marsh.

Fenestrated Refers to a type of leaf anatomy with small perforation or transparent spots.

Fermentation The process of growing microorganisms within an enclosed tank called as fermenter, under controlled conditions of aeration, agitation, temperature, and pH.

Fermenter Refers to a tank or vessel used for carrying out fermentation.

Ferredoxin A protein containing more than one iron and acid-labile sulfur, which displays electron-transfer activity but not classical enzyme function.

Ferric chloride (alcoholic) Used for the detection of phenols.

Ferriheme Refers to an iron(III) porphyrin coordination complex.

Ferritin An iron storage protein consisting of a shell of 24 protein subunits and encapsulating up to 4500 iron atoms in the form of a hydrated iron(III) oxide.

Ferrochelatase An enzyme that catalyzes the insertion of iron into protoporphyrin IX to form heme.

Ferroheme Refers to an iron(II) porphyrin coordination complex.

Fertilization The process by which the haploid male gamete and female gamete fuse to produce a diploid zygote.

Fertilizer Used for describing any substance which is applied to increase soil fertility and consequent increase in plant growth that may be organic or inorganic. Main fertilizers are nitrate, potash and phosphates. Relative amount of these are expressed in N:P:K ratios.

Fetal calf serum The liquid portion that remains after natural coagulation of blood drawn from the heart of an unborn calf.

Fever A human body temperature above the normal 98.4°F (37°C). Also known as pyrexia.

Fiber Elongated and thickened cell found in xylem tissue, which strengthens and supports the surrounding cells.

Fiber tracheid A fiber with thick walls and pointed ends which has simple pits and is found in wood tissue.

Fibrin Refers to a plasma protein which in its aggregated state, is the major component of a blood clot. It is produced from fibrinogen, which is a soluble precursor, by the action of the proteolytic enzyme, thrombin.

Fibrinogen Also known as factor I in the clotting of blood. The plasma protein becomes converted to a clot at the end of the coagulation process, present in plasma and absent in serum.

Fibroblast The type of cell that usually lives in the dermis and produces collagen molecules in that location.

Fibromyalgia Refers to a symptom complex of fatigue, muscle aches, and tender spots in different areas of the body.

Fibrous cortex Of lichens, having a cortex that is made up of hypae lying parallel with the longitudinal axis of the thallus.

Fibrous root A root system found in monocot plants in that branches develop from the adventitious roots, forming a system in which all roots are about the same size and length.

Filament Refers to the stalk bearing the anther.

Filgrastim Filgrastim is an *Escherichia coli*-derived glycoprotein.

Filiform Thread-like, long and slender.

Film-coated tablets Film-coated tablets are compressed tablets that are coated with a thin layer of a water-insoluble or water-soluble polymer, (e.g. hydroxypropyl methylcellulose, ethylcellulose, povidone, PEG).

Filtration Removal of suspended matter from a fluid by passing it through a porous medium which prevents particles from getting through, usually by entrapment on or in the filter matrix.

Fimbrial Refers to leaf venation, veins joining and forming a continuous vein running just inside the margin of the blade.

Final bulk product The final drug product that is ready for concentration, drying, and filling into containers prior to dispensing and final filling, after chemical or biological processing and purification.

Finished product A medicinal product which has undergone all stages of production, including packaging in its final container.

First law of thermodynamics (conservation) Energy is neither created nor destroyed, it changes from one form to another.

First time effects First time effects (presystemic elimination) occur with drugs given orally. A portion of the drug is eliminated before systemic absorption occurs.

Fischer projection Refers to a projection formula in which vertically drawn bonds are considered to lie under the projection plane and horizontal bonds to lie over that plane.

Fissile material A radioisotope which could undergo a nuclear fission reaction and is frequently found at reactor sites or as part of a nuclear weapon.

Fistular Hollow all through its length.

Fixation The process in which the internal and external structures of cells are preserved and fixed in position.

Fixed oils and fats Glyceryl esters of fatty acids which are saponifiable by alkalies. Liquid at normal temperature is fixed oil, while those that are semisolid or solid are known as fats.

Flaccid Weak, soft, or flabby. Leaves which do not have enough water and are about to wilt or are wilting.

Flag leaf Refers to the leaf immediately below the inflorescence.

Flagellin The protein that is used to construct the filament of a bacterial flagellum.

Flaggelae Refers to thin, helical filaments that are attached to the surface of bacterial and eukaryotic cells. They are motile structures containing microtubules (composed of proteins called tubulin) that allow cells possessing them to move.

Flammable liquid Refers to any liquid having a closed cup flash point below 100°F (37.8°C). They do not comprise compressed gases or cryogenic fluids.

Flammable solid A solid substance, other than one which is defined as a blasting agent or explosive, which is liable to cause fire through friction or as a result of retained heat from manufacture, that has an ignition temperature below 212°F (100°C), or which burns so vigorously when ignited that it creates a serious hazard. These include finely divided solid materials that when dispersed in air as a cloud could be ignited and cause an explosion.

Flash vacuum pyrolysis (FVP) Thermal reaction of a molecule by exposing it to a short thermal shock at high temperature and generally in the gas phase.

Flatulence Refers to gas in the stomach or intestines.

Flavanones Flavonoids isomeric with chalcones, differing from flavones in lacking the double bond in the 2,3: position. They are usually colorless or slightly yellow.

Flavedo Outer part of the rind of citrus fruit that bears oil glands and pigments.

Flavin A prosthetic group which is found in flavoproteins and is involved in biological oxidation and reduction.

Flavones Refers to flavonoids which lack the 3:hydroxy group of flavonols and is derived from flavanones by oxidation, yellow in color.

Flavonoids Refers to a C:15 skeleton with a chroman ring bearing an aromatic ring in position 2, 3, or 4. There are two benzene rings in the flavonoid nucleus, one derived from condensation of acetate units (three malonyl units), the other derived from the shikimic acid pathway (cinnamic acid), and these are joined by a C3 structure that may be open or closed. The flavonoid nucleus is usually attached to a sugar, forming a water soluble glycoside.

Flavonols The flavonoids differ from flavones in having a 3-hydroxyl substituent. They are yellow color pigments.

Flavour Flavour is the sensory impression of a food or other substance. It is determined by the three chemical senses of taste, olfaction (smell), and trigeminal senses that detect chemical irritants in the mouth and throat.

Floc Mass having a feathery or wooly appearance.

Flocculation A technique for the separation of liquid/solids. Cationic or anionic polyelectrolytes are added to highly colloidal water causing coagulation and subsequent settling.

Flora Plants found in a particular area and also, a publication listing and (usually) describing the species of plants found in a particular area.

Floral cup Refers to hypanthium.

Floral diagram An useful plan diagram of flowers showing their general orientation and the number and relationships (aestivation, connation, adnation, etc.) of their parts.

Floral formula A formula referring the number and some of the relationships (connation, adnation, etc.) of the parts of a flower.

Floret Refers to an individual flower in a grass spikelet.

Floricane Refers to the stem at flowering and fruiting stage.

Flow cytometry Analysis of biological material by detectig the light-absorbing or fluorescing properties of cells or subcellular fractions (i.e. chromosomes) passing in a narrow stream through a laser beam.

Flow decay Measuring the decline in flow rate through a filter to found a silt index for the water being filtered. This silt index is a measure of suspended solids and their ability to clog the filter.

Flow restrictor Flow-limiting orifice used to control flow rate in a liquid stream.

Flower Refers to the part of a plant containing or consisting of the organs of reproduction, either together in a monoclinous flower or separate in male and female flowers.

Flower bud Refers to a bud in which contain flower parts.

Flower essences Flower essences are made by infusing flowers in water and then adding alcohol as a preservative. These essences are used internally or topically to balance emotional states and the underlying philosophy focuses on stabilizing emotions in order to drive away illness and stimulate internal healing processes.

Flu-like symptoms Refers to series of symptoms that may include fever, muscle aches, chills, headaches and fatigue.

Fluid extract A liquid extract of raw plant material(s), generally of a concentration ratio of 1 part raw herb to 1 part solvent (1:1). Fluidextracts contain alcohol as a solvent, preservative, or both.

Fluidized bed A container that is holding powder coating material which is aerated from below so as to form an air-supported expanded cloud of such material through which the preheated object to be coated is immersed and transported.

Fluorescein Refers to an orange-red compound, $C_{20}H_{12}O_5$ that exhibits intense fluorescence in alkaline solution.

Fluorescence microscope A microscope which exposes a specimen to light of a specific wavelength and then forms an image from the fluorescent light produced.

Fluorinated plastics Fluorinated plastics are thermoplastic paraffinic polymers where the hydrogen has been replaced by fluorine.

Fluxional A fluxional chemical species undergoes rapid rearrangements, usually detectable by methods which observe the behaviour of individual nuclei in a rearranged chemical species.

Folate coenzymes Refers to a group of heterocyclic compounds which are based on the 4-(2-amino-3,4-dihydro-4-oxopteridin-6-ylmethylamino) benzoic acid (pteroic acid) and conjugated with one or more L-glutamate units. Folate derivatives are significant in DNA synthesis and erythrocyte formation and deficiency of folate leads to anemia.

Foliaceous That has the form or texture of a foliage leaf, also thin and leaf-like.

Folium Refers to the leaf of plant.

Follicle-stimulating hormone (FSH) A hormone secreted by the anterior pituitary which promotes gamete formation in males and females.

Fomentation A technique in which we apply a warm and moist cloth, soaked in an infusion or decoction, as treatment.

Food chain Flow of energy and matter in living organisms through a producer-consumer series.

Food intoxication Food poisoning caused by microbial toxins produced in a food prior to consumption and also it purely does not indicates the presence of living bacteria.

Food poisoning Term referring to a gastrointestinal disease caused by eating the food contaminated by pathogens or their toxins.

Forb Refers to a non-woody plant other than a grass, sedge, or rush.

Formaldehyde Refers to a colorless, highly irritating, pungent compound used in the pharmaceutical and cosmetic industries.

Formic acid A colorless, volatile acid that irritates skin.

Formulary A pre-determined list of drugs and medications.

Formulation development Formulation development is a continuing process. Initial drug formulations are developed for early clinical studies. When the submission of an NDA is considered, the manufacturer attempts to develop the final (marketed) dosage form. The dose of the drug and the route of administration are important in determining the modifications needed.

Forward flow test An objective and quantitative method of determining filter integrity in which the filter is wetted and a predetermined constant air pressure is applied. A measurement is made for pure diffusional airflow through the wetted membrane. If the diffusional airflow across the membrane is below the maximum permissible value given, then the filter is suitable.

Fossil Refers to an impression of plant part in earth's crust.

Fossil alkali Refers to sodium carbonate.

Fossil fuels Fuels which are formed in the earth from plant or animal residues, e.g. coal, petroleum and natural gas.

Fouling Happens when gelatinous coatings, colloidal masses or dense bacterial growth form a compacted coating on membrane or filter surfaces which blocks further flow.

Fragmentation Production of new individuals from fragments of original individual.

Frass Solid fecal material that is produced by insects.

Free electron Electron that is not attached to a nucleus.

Free energy The energy of a system which is available to do work at constant temperature and pressure.

Free radical A free radical, oxidant or oxidizer or oxidizing agent, is a molecule with one extra electron which wants to take an electron away from another molecule and use that electron to stabilize itself. This process damages (oxidizes) many biological chemicals including the lipids in cell membranes and are the causative agents for various diseases.

Free rotation The rotation about a bond is called free when the rotational barrier is so low that different conformations are not perceptible as different chemical species on the time scale of the experiment.

Freeze drying Technique in which plant materials are frozen, then subjected to high vacuum, water molecules sublimate (pass from solid to gas phase), and are removed from the material.

Freezing point The freezing point, or melting point, of a pure compound is the temperature at which the solid and the liquid phases are in equilibrium under a pressure of 1 atmosphere (atm). The freezing point of a solution is the temperature at which the solid phase of the pure solvent and the liquid phase of the solution are in equilibrium under a pressure of 1 atm.

Frequency of medicine The number of times each day that a medication is administered. Fresh weight: Similar as wet weight.

Fructans Refers to polysaccharides derived from fructose.

Fructose Refers to a hexose sugar forming a 5-membered ring.

Fruit The developed ovary of the flower containing ripe seeds, whether fleshy or dry.

Fruiting body A particular structure that holds sexually or asexually produced spores, which is found in fungi and in some bacteria.

Frustule Refers to siliceous cell wall of a diatom.

Frutescent Becoming shrub-like.

Fucoidan Refers to water-soluble, sulfated polysaccharide in Phaeophycean cell wall.

Fucoxanthin Brown pigment that is found in and characteristic of the brown algae.

Fume hoods Parts which collect fumes from chemicals, solvents, acids, and other hazardous materials. Hoods may include HEPA filters if powders are present, or carbon filters to filter fumes from the work surface and most fume hoods are 100% exhausted to outdoors.

Fumigation Treatment of materials with a pesticide active ingredient that is a gas under treatment conditions.

Functional foods Foods that have components or ingredient incorporated in them to give them a specific medical or physiological benefit other than a purely nutritional effect.

Functional group Generally organic compounds are considered as consisting of a relatively unreactive backbone, e.g. a chain of sp^3 hybridized carbon atoms, and one or several functional groups. The functional group is an atom, or a group of atoms which have similar chemical properties whenever it occurs in different compounds and it defines the characteristic physical and chemical properties of families of organic compounds. Examples includes alcohol group-OH, amine group-NH_2, etc.

Functional gene tests Biochemical assays for a specific protein, which indicates that a specific gene is not just present but active.

Fungi Low forms of plant life unable to form carbohydrates and protein that are widespread in nature. Fungal cells are larger than bacterial cells, and their characteristic internal structures, like nucleus and vacuoles, can be seen easily with a light microscope. Its body usually consists of filamentous strands called mycelium and reproduces through dispersal of spores. Based upon their mode of sexual reproduction, fungi are grouped in four classes, phycomycetes, ascomycetes, deuteromycetes and basidiomycetes. Yeasts and molds are the two major groups of fungi.

Fungicide A pesticide used for control of fungi or an agent that kills fungi.

Fungistatic An agent that inhibits the growth and reproduction of fungi.

Funicle Refers to the stalk of an ovule.

Furanocoumarins Refers to group of complex coumarins in which the coumarin structure is prenylated.

Fusion The process of melting together or fusing together into one.

Fusion welding Refers to welding in that the base material is fused together without the addition of filler material to the weld.

G

Galactans Term used for describing hemicellulose, mucilages pectins and gums that yield galactose on hydrolysis.

Galactoaraban Refers to a polysaccharide that is a polymer having galactose and arabinose.

Galactogogue Agent that increases breast milk secretion.

Galactopyranose Refers to the pyranose form of galactose which on prolymerisation forms the hemicellulose galactan.

Galactose A hexose sugar that is commonly found in plants.

Galactosidase Refers to an enzyme that catalyses the hydrolysis of galactosides.

Galacturonic acid Term used for the acid formed from galactose and these units are condensed to form pectic acid, which reacts with calcium or magnesium to form insoluble pectates.

Gallic acid It is a type of hydrolyzable tannin.

Gametophyte A phase in the life history producing gamete.

Gametangium Cell in which gametes are formed.

Gametes Term refers to haploid reproductive cells, ovum and sperm.

Gamma globulin A blood protein which plays a major role in the process of immunity. Sometimes also refers to a whole group of blood proteins that are known as antibodies or immunoglobulins (Ig). Mostly, it applies to a particular immunoglobulin, designated as IgG, which is believed to be the most abundant type of antibody in the body.

Gamopetalous Having the petals united so as to form a tube-like corolla.

Ganglia Clusters of neurons, which receive and process signals.

Gas gangrene A type of gangrene which arises from dirty, lacerated wounds infected by anaerobic bacteria, especially species of Clostridium and as the bacteria grow, they release toxins and ferment carbohydrates to produce carbon dioxide and hydrogen gas.

Gas room A separately ventilated, fully enclosed room in that only toxic and highly toxic compressed gases and associated equipment and supplies are stored or used.

Gas vacuole A gas filled vacuole which is found in cyanobacteria and some other aquatic bacteria that provides flotation and is composed of gas vesicles that are made of protein.

Gas-phase acidity The negative of the Gibbs energy change for the reaction.

Gas-phase basicity The negative of the Gibbs energy change associated with the reaction.

Gastrin A hormone produced by the pyloric gland area of the stomach which stimulates the secretion of gastric acids.

Gastritis Inflammation of the stomach.

Gastroenteritis An acute inflammation of the lining of the stomach and intestines, that is characterized by anorexia, nausea, diarrhea, abdominal pain, and weakness. The causes includes food poisoning due to organisms like *E. coli*, *S. aureus*, Campylobacter and Salmonella species or consumption of irritating food or drink, or psychological factors such as anger, stress and fear.

GCP Good clinical practice.

Geiger counter Instrument which measures radiation output.

Gel A colloid in which the dispersed phase is liquid and the dispersion medium is solid.

Gel electrophoresis A DNA separation technique which is very important in DNA sequencing that involves cloning DNA fragments into special sequencing cloning vectors that carry tiny pieces of DNA and the next step is to determine the base sequence of the tiny fragments by a special procedure that generates a series of even tinier DNA fragments that differ in size by only one base. Finally, these nested fragments are separated by gel electrophoresis, in which the DNA pieces are added to a gelatinous solution, allowing the fragments to work their way down through the gel. Pieces that are small move faster and will reach the bottom first. By applying an electrical field to the gel movement through the gel is accelerated.

Gelatin A protein formed from the collagen of the tissues by boiling in water.

Gene One of the units of inherited material which is carried on a chromosome, arranged in a linear fashion and are indivisible, but capable of self-replication. Each gene represents a unit character that has been recognized by its effect on the individual bearing the gene in its cells. In each nucleus, there are 1000 genes. Genes are also discrete segments of DNA that contain the genetic code.

Gene expression It is the process by which a gene's coded information is converted into the structures present and operating in the cell. The expressed genes include those which are transcribed into mRNA and then translated into protein and those which are transcribed into RNA but not translated into protein.

Gene family Refers to group of closely related genes which makes similar products.

Gene gun A device which uses high-pressure gas or another propellant to discharge a spray of DNA-coated microprojectiles into cells and transform them.

Gene mapping Determination of the relative positions of genes on a DNA molecule and of the distance, in linkage units, between them.

Gene product The biochemical material, either RNA or protein that results from expression of a gene. Its amount is used to measure how active a gene is and abnormal amounts can be correlated with disease causing alleles.

Gene sequencing Determination of the sequence of bases in a DNA strand. The two most widely used methods are the chain-termination method and the chemical method.

Gene splicing Refers to the enzymatic attachment of one gene or part of a gene to another.

Gene therapy Insertion of normal DNA directly into cells to correct a generic defect is referred as gene therapy.

Genera Taxonomic subcategories within families, composed of one or more species, singular: genus.

General recombination Recombination involves a reciprocal exchange of a pair of homologous DNA sequences and it can occur at any place on the chromosome.

Generalized transduction The transfer of any part of a genome when the DNA fragment is packaged within a phage capsid by mistake.

Generation time The time required for a microbial population to double in number.

Generic drug A drug produced and marketed under its chemical or generic name (e.g. paracetamol) as opposed to calpol, a brand name for the former. A generic drug can be sold only after a proprietary drug goes off patent. Though generic drugs are cheaper for consumers, they still must meet the standards of GMPs as set out by the FDA. A generic drug product is therapeutically equivalent to the brand name drug product and contains the same amount of the drug in the same type of dosage form, (e.g. tablets, liquids, injectables). It must be bioequivalent, (i.e. have the same rate and extent of drug absorption) to the brand drug product. Therefore, a generic drug product is expected to give the same clinical response. These studies are normally performed with healthy human volunteers.

It may differ from the brand product in physical appearance, (i.e. size, color, shape) or in the amount and type of excipients only for tablets. It may not differ in both the qualitative and quantitative compositions for liquids, injectables, semisolids, transdermals, inhalation, products, and optical products unless adequate safety studies have been performed.

Genetic code Refers to the sequence of nucleotides, coded in triplets (codons) along the mRNA which determines the sequence of amino acids in protein synthesis. The DNA sequence of a gene could be used to predict the mRNA sequence and the genetic code could in turn be used to predict the amino acid sequence.

Genetic diseases Diseases which occur because of a mutation in the genetic material.

Genetic drug substitution Genetic drug substitution is the process of dispensing a genetic drug product in place of the prescribed drug product, (e.g. generic product for brand name product, generic product for another generic product, brand name product for generic product). The substituted product must be a therapeutic equivalent to the prescribed product.

Genetic engineering The selective, purposeful alteration of genes by technological means.

Genetics The scientific study of heredity that involves how particular qualities or traits are transmitted from parents to offspring. It deals with the study of its chemical foundation, its developmental expression and its bearing on variation, selection adaptation, evolution breeding and the activities of man.

Genome Refers to a complete set of haploid number of chromosomes there in an organism.

Genomic library A collection of clones prepared from a set of randomly generated overlapping DNA fragments that represents the entire genome of an organism.

Genomic sequence The order of the subunits, called bases which makes up a particular fragment of DNA in a genome.

Geno type The genetic composition of an organism that includes expressed and nonexpressed genes, which may not be readily apparent.

Genus A taxonomic group consisting of closely related species. These genera are being grouped into families.

Geophyte Plants with an underground dormant part like tuber, bulb, rhizome, etc. to help the plant survive adverse conditions.

Geotropism The directional growth response (tropism) of a plant or part of a plant to gravity. For example, roots grow downward, showing positive geotropism, while shoots grow upward in a negative response.

Germicidal lamps Light sources which emit ultraviolet radiation at a wavelength of 254 nanometers (nm), commonly found in biological safety cabinets and used to inactivate bacteria, viruses and fungi which are either air-borne or on exposed surfaces.

Germicide An agent that destroys microorganisms.

Germifuge That expels germs.

Germination The process by which the embryo restarts growth and escapes from the limitations of the seed or fruit and formation of the young sporophyte (seedling).

Germplasm The total genetic variability, represented by germ cells or seeds, which is available to a particular population of organisms or an individual, group of individuals. Otherwise known as a clone representing a genotype, variety, species or culture, held in an *in situ* or *ex situ* collection.

Ghon complex Refers to the initial focus of parenchymal infection in primary pulmonary tuberculosis.

Giardiasis A common intestinal disease that is caused by the parasitic protozoan, *Giardia lamblia*.

Gibberellins Growth hormones which accelerates shoot growth. Gibberellins were first discovered in the fungus *Gibberella fujikuroi*, and later on in other plants.

Gibbous Of shape, a distended, rounded swelling on one side, as on a calyx or corolla tube or segment.

Gingivitis Inflammation of the gums surrounding teeth.

Girdle Damage which completely encircles a stem or root, more frequently resulting in death of plant parts above or below the girdle.

Glabrous With a smooth, even surface or without hairs.

Glacial Glass-like, crystallized.

Gland Refers to a secreting part or appendage.

Glandular Having secreting organs, glands or trichomes.

Glauber's salt Refers to sodium sulfate, $Na_2SO_4 \cdot 10H_2O$.

Glaucous Refers to colour, blueish or whitish green in colour, with a whitish bloom.

Gliding motility Refers to a type of motility in that a microbial cell glides along when in contact with a solid surface.

Gliding movement Movement of an organism when in contact with substratum.

Globose Of shape, rounded, almost spherical, globular.

Globulin A type of blood protein which is elevated in systemic inflammatory diseases like lupus erythematosus and rheumatoid arthritis. The antibody molecules are a form of globulin protein.

Glomerulonephritis An inflammatory disease of the renal glomeruli.

Glucagon A hormone, which is released by the pancreas that stimulates the breakdown of glycogen and the release of glucose, thereby increasing blood levels of glucose. Glucagon and insulin work together to maintain the sugar levels in blood.

Glucans Polysaccharides composed of glucose units held together by glycosidic linkages.

Glucocorticoids A group of steroid hormones produced by the adrenal cortex which are important in regulating the metabolism of carbohydrates, fats and proteins.

Gluconeogenesis Term refers to the synthesis of glucose from noncarbohydrate precursors such as lactate and amino acids.

Glucose A hexose sugar forming a six-membered ring.

Glucoside A glycoside that has glucose as its sugar unit is called a glucoside.

Glucosinolates Mustard oil glycosides, mostly colorless, with a sharp, odor that through hydrolysis with myrosine yield isothiocyanates or mustard oils.

Glucuronic acid The type of luronic acid that is derived from glucose and is a common constituent of gums and mucilages.

Glutathione A water-soluble antioxidant which is found in onions and potatoes that may detoxify cancer-causing substances. Also it supports the actions of other antioxidants, such as vitamins C and E and beta carotene.

Gluten A reserve protein that is found in plants that causes dough to be sticky.

Glutinous Having a sticky, moist surface, a gluey or sticky exudation.

Glycoalkaloid A compound containing nitrogen in the heterocyclic ring and a sugar part.

Glycocalyx A network of polysaccharides that extends from the surface of bacteria and other cells.

Glycoflavones Refers to class of flavonoids that have a sugar attached.

Glycogen A complex carbohydrate which is the main form in which glucose is stored in the body, mainly in the liver and muscles.

Glycolipids Polysaccharides formed of sugars linked to lipids, which is a part of the cell membrane.

Glycolysis The anaerobic conversion of glucose to lactic acid by using the Embden-Meyerhof pathway.

Glycoproteins Refer to polysaccharides formed of sugars linked to proteins. On the outer surface of a membrane, these glycoproteins act as receptors for molecular signals originating outside the cell.

Glycoside Compounds containing a sugar component (glycone) and a nonsugar (aglycone) component which on hydrolysis yields one or more sugars.

Glyoxylate cycle It is a modified tricarboxylic acid cycle in which the decarboxylation reactions are bypassed by the enzymes isocitrate lyase and malate synthase. It is mainly used to convert acetyl-CoA to succinate and other metabolites.

GMP (good manufacturing practice) GMP ensures that pharmaceutical products are manufactured consistently and are controlled to the specific standards of quality. To be GMP certified, a company must show that its facilities and equipment are appropriate, its staff has the required levels of training, and that it manufactures according to approved procedures, maintains detailed manufacturing records and follows the regulatory norms on storage and transport.

GMP critical parameter Refers to a parameter that has a direct effect on product quality.

Gnetales Group of seed plants restricted to three genera (*Gnetum*, *Ephedra*, and *Welwitschia*).

Gnotobiotic Animals which are microorganism free or live in association with one or more known microorganisms.

Gold drugs Gold coordination compounds that are used in the treatment of rheumatoid arthritis, examples being auranofin.

Golgi bodies Very small particles that are composed of membrane

aggregates and are responsible for the secretion of certain enzymes and macromolecules. They are the deposition and packaging site for many excreted products.

Golgi apparatus A membranous eucaryotic organelle which is composed of stacks of flattened sacs (cisternae) and is involved in packaging and modifying materials for secretion and many other processes.

Gonadotropins Hormones that are produced by the anterior pituitary that affect the testis and ovary, which include follicle-stimulating hormone and luteinizing hormone.

Gonococci Bacteria of the species *Neisseria gonorrhoeae* and this is the organism causing gonorrhea.

Gonorrhea An acute infectious sexually transmitted disease, caused by *Neisseria gonorrhoeae*, of the mucous membranes of the genitourinary tract, eye, rectum, and throat.

Gossypetin Refers to 8: hydroxy-flavonoid, a yellow flavonoid.

Gossypol A substance that is poisonous to many animals, produced by numerous small glands in most cotton varieties.

Gout A metabolic condition, which is characterized by painful inflammation of the joints caused by excess uric acid in the blood.

Graft Refers to a part of a plant, stem or root, inserted into and/or fusing with, another, usually referring to different plants, whether of the same or different species.

Graft hybrid A chimaera produced by grafting dissimilar plants.

Graft-versus-host disease A disease that results when mature post-thymic T cells in donor grafts (e.g. bone marrow) identify the host as foreign and attack it.

Grain In general refers to, any small, rounded structure.

Gram-negative bacteria Refers to bacteria, which lose violet colour on staining with a basic dye like gentician violet and mordant when they are subsequently made to treat with a decolouring agent and readily take up red colour when counter stained with a red dye, e.g. neutral red. These bacteria are less susceptible to antibiotics. Examples, includes *Escherichia coli*, *Salmonella*, and other Enterobacteriaceae, *Pseudomonas*, *Moraxella*, *Helicobacter*, *Stenotrophomonas*, *Bdellovibrio*, etc.

Gram-positive bacteria Refers to bacteria, which retain violet colour on staining with a basic dye and mordant even after treatment by decolourizing agent and counter staining with red dye. These bacteria are more susceptible to antibiotic detergents. It includes many well-known genera such as *Bacillus*, *Listeria*, *Staphylococcus*, *Streptococcus*, *Enterococcus* and *Clostridium*.

Gram stain A differential staining procedure that divides bacteria into gram-positive and gram-negative groups based on their ability to retain crystal violet when decolorized with an organic solvent like ethanol.

Granuloma Term applied to nodular inflammatory lesions containing phagocytic cells.

Green algae Term used for describing members of division Chlorophyta. They are green pigmented having mainly chlorophyll, store starch as food reserve and the cell wall is made up of cellulose mainly.

Green house gases Gases released from the earth's surface through chemical and biological processes, which interact with the chemicals in the stratosphere to decrease the release of radiation from the earth, which is believed to be the cause of global warming.

Green manure Any fast-growing, inexpensive crop sown towards the end of season is ploughed into the soil when it is green so that it may increase soil organic matter on decomposition.

Green salt Refers to uranium(IV) fluoride, UF_4.

Grippe An antiquated term that refers for influenza or an epidemic cold.

Griselinoside Refers to iridoid glucoside.

Ground meristem Apical meristem of stem or root, producing cortex and pith.

Ground tissue Refers to the tissues other than the epidermis, periderm and vascular tissue.

Growth chamber A chamber, which is used for the incubation of culture containers or plants under controlled conditions.

Growth An increase in cellular constituents.

Growth factors Organic compounds, which must be supplied in the diet for growth because they are essential cell components or precursors of such components and they cannot be synthesized by the organism.

Growth hormone A peptide hormone that is produced by the anterior pituitary that is essential for growth.

Growth rings Refers to the features of woody stems produced by plants growing in areas with seasonal (as opposed to year-long) growth. The growth ring marks the position of the vascular cambium at the end of the previous year's growth.

Guanine A purine derivative, 2-amino-6-oxypurine, which is found in nucleosides, nucleotides and nucleic acids.

Guanylate cyclase An enzyme that catalyzes the conversion of guanosine 5'-triphosphate to cyclic guanosine 3',5'-monophosphate that is involved in cellular regulation processes.

Guard cells Pair of cells that surround a stomate and regulate its size by altering their shape.

Gumma A soft, gummy tumor occurring in tertiary syphilis.

Gums Refers to complex water soluble polysaccharides that exudates from branches.

Gut-associated lymphoid tissue (GALT) The defensive lymphoid tissue, which is present in the intestines.

Guttation Formation of water drops on plants from moisture in air. Also the process of water being exuded from hydathodes at the enlarged terminations of veins around the margins of the leaves.

Gymnosperm Refers to plants that produces seeds that are not enclosed. This includes any seed plant that does not produce flowers.

Gynaecium The female organs of the flower that consists of one or more carpels forming one or several ovaries with their stigmas and styles.

Gynocardin Refers to a cyclopentenoid cyanogenic glycoside.

Gynophore Refers to a stalk that supports ovary.

H

Habit Refers to the external look or way of growth of a plant, e.g. climbing, erect, bushy, etc.

Habitat Refers to the area or external environment in which a plant lives.

Habitat form A plant that shows features, which are abnormal, but it can be related to the place where it is growing, e.g. retarded growth under poor conditions.

Habituation Refers to the process by which an organism gets accustomed to the new environmental conditions.

Haem Term used for one of a group of iron-porphyrins that get conjugated with proteins to form peroxidase, catalase and the cytochromes.

HAI Health Action International.

Hair Refers to any elongate single or multicelled glandular or nonglandular outgrowth from the epidermis.

Hairpin A double helical area formed by base pairing between adjacent complementary sequences in a single strand of RNA or DNA.

Half-life The amount of time a drug takes for half of its initial amount to disintegrate. In a kinetic experiment, the time required for the concentration of a particular reacting species to fall to one-half of its initial value.

Half-chair Refers to the conformation of a six-membered ring structure in which four contiguous atoms are in a plane and the other two atoms lie on opposite sides of the plane is called a half-chair.

Halobacteria A group of archaea, which have an absolute dependence on high NaCl concentrations for growth and will not survive at a concentration below about 1.5 M NaCl, also known as extreme halophiles.

Halochromism This refers to the colour change that occurs on addition of acid (or base, or a salt) to a solution of a compound.

Haloenzyme Refers to an enzyme which contains a non-protein component.

Halogen Refers to one of the chlorine group (bromine, chlorine, fluorine, iodine) of elements, all being univalent. They form monobasic acids with hydrogen, and their hydroxides are monobasic acids.

Haloperoxidase A peroxidase that catalyzes the oxidative transformation of halides to XO^- (X being Cl, Br or I), or organic halogen compounds in which, most are hemeproteins, but some bromoperoxidases from algae are vanadium-containing enzymes .

Halophile Refers to an organism, which displays accelerated growth or is dependent on high salt concentrations or a microorganism that requires high levels of sodium chloride for growth.

Halophyte Refers to any species, which is capable of tolerating 0.5% or more NaCl.

Handedness This term has been used in either ways, chirality or chirality sense.

Hansch analysis It is the investigation of the quantitative relationship between the biological activity of a series of compounds and their physicochemical substituent or global parameters representing hydrophobic, electronic, steric and other effects using multiple regression correlation methodology.

Hantavirus pulmonary syndrome Refers to the disease in humans whicah is caused by the pulmonary syndrome hantavirus. When humans inhale the virus, first develop ordinary flu-like aches and pains, within few days the hantavirus causes lung damage and capillary leakage and after about a week the infected person enters a crisis phase and may die.

Haplo (prefix) Having a single set of something.

Haploid A single set of chromosomes, which is present in the egg and sperm cells of animals and in the egg and pollen cells of plants. In the reproductive cells of human beings, there are 23 chromosomes.

Haplostele It is a variant of a protostele in which the phloem surrounds the xylem.

Hapten A molecule which is not immunogenic by itself but that, when coupled to a macromolecular carrier it can elicit antibodies directed against itself.

Harborage transmission Refers to the mode of transmission in that an infectious organism does not undergo morphological or physiological changes within the vector.

Hard acid A Lewis acid with an acceptor centre of low polarizability, preferentially associates with hard bases rather than with soft bases, in a qualitative sense. On the contrary, a soft acid possesses an acceptor centre of high polarizability and exhibits the reverse preference for a partner for coordination.

Hard base A Lewis base with a donor centre of low polarizability and the reverse applies to soft bases.

Hard drug A hard drug is a compound which is nonmetabolizable, characterized either by high lipid solubility and accumulation in adipose tissues and organelles, or by high water solubility.

Hardness Of water, refers to concentration of calcium and magnesium salts in water.

Harvesting Of biotechnology refres to the separation of cells from growth media which can be accomplished by filtration, precipitation, or centrifugation. When it comes to the plants, refers to separation of required parts.

Hastate Of shape, shaped, more or less triangular with the two basal lobes divergent.

Hay fever Also, allergic rhinitis, a type of atopic allergy involving the upper respiratory tract.

Hazardous chemical reaction A reaction that generates pressure or byproducts and which could cause injury, illness or harm to humans, domestic animals, or wildlife.

Hazardous substance A substance because of being explosive, flammable, toxic, poisonous, corrosive, oxidizing, irritant or otherwise harmful, is likely to cause injury.

Haze Refers to the appearance of a localized diminishing in brightness or shine of a surface when compared to the neighboring surfaces.

Health hazard Categorization of a chemical for which there is evidence based and established scientific principles that acute or chronic health effects may occur in exposed persons. The health hazards include chemicals that are carcinogens, toxic or highly toxic agents, reproductive toxins, irritants, corrosives, sensitizers, hepatotoxins, nephrotoxins, neurotoxins, agents that act on the hematopoietic system, and agents that damage the lungs, skin, eyes or mucous membranes.

Healing touch It is a type of practice, practiced by registered nurses and others to accelerate wound healing, relieve pain, promote relaxation, prevent illness and ease the dying process. The practitioner uses light touch or works with their hands near the client's body in an effort to restore balance to the client's energy system.

Health A state of optimal physical, mental, and social well-being, and not merely indicates the absence of disease and illness.

Healthy carrier Refers to any individual who harbors a pathogen, but is not ill.

Heartwood The dead inner portion of the xylem (wood) of a trunk or large root.

Heat-labile Compouds which are able to be destroyed or altered by high temperature. In the process of sterilization, heat labile pharmaceuticals are sterilized by filtration.

Heat-shock proteins Refers to those proteins which are produced when cells are exposed to high temperatures or other stressful conditions. These proteins protect the cells from damage and often aid in the proper folding of proteins.

Heat of vaporization The amount of heat required to change a unit volume from a liquid to a vapor at a given pressure without a change in temperature.

Heavy metals They are high molecular weight metal ions, like lead.

Hela cells Human cervical carcinoma cells used to study the biochemistry and genetics of human cell growth.

Helical In virology, refers to a virus with a helical capsid surrounding its nucleic acid.

Helicases Enzymes which use ATP energy to unwind DNA ahead of the replication fork.

Helicity Refers to the chirality of a helical, propeller or screw-shaped molecular unit. The right-handed helix is described as P or plus and a left-handed one as M or minus.

Helix A spiral, staircase-like, arrangement with a repeating pattern described by two simultaneous operations, rotation, and translation and also it is the natural conformation of many biological polymers.

Helper T cells A type of lymphocyte, which stimulates the production of antibodies by activating B cells when an antigen is present.

Hemadsorption The adherence of red blood cells to the surface of something, like another cell or a virus.

Hemagglutination Refers to the agglutination of red blood cells by antibodies.

Hemagglutinin The antibody which is responsible for a hemagglutination reaction.

Hematin An iron protoporphyrin, which differs from heme in that the central iron atom is in the ferric (Fe^{+++}) rather than the ferrous (Fe^{++}) state.

Hemerythrin A dioxygen-carrying protein from marine invertebrates that contains an oxo-bridged dinuclear iron center.

Hemicellulose Matrix of polysaccharides that contains galactose, xylose, etc. and cross-linking cellulose molecules.

Hemochromatosis Refers to a genetic condition, characterized by massive iron overload leading to cirrhosis and/or other tissue damage, attributable to iron.

Hemoflagellate A flagellated protozoan parasite which is found in the bloodstream.

Hemoglobin The red, respiratory conjugated protein of erythrocytes, which consists of approximately 6% heme and 94% globin (a protein).

Hemolysin A substance which causes hemolysis (the lysis of red blood cells).

Hemolysis The disruption of red blood cells and release of their hemoglobin.

Hemolytic uremic syndrome A kidney disease, which is characterized by blood in the urine and often by kidney failure.

Hemophilia A hereditary, plasma-coagulation disorder, mainly affecting males but transmitted by females, and are characterized by excessive, sometimes spontaneous, bleeding.

Hemopoietic Pertains to or related to the formation of blood cells.

Hemorrhagic fever A fever that is typically caused by a specific virus that may lead to hemorrhage, shock, and sometimes death.

Hemostatic An agent, which is used to stop internal bleeding.

HEPA (high efficiency particulate air) filters They are filters with a minimum efficiency of 99.97% for 0.3 µm particle size as determined by test. They are made of compressed and bonded microfiber glass or Teflon® corrugated to produce a high surface area in a small area panel of filter medium. When operated at design velocity, larger and smaller particles are captured at higher efficiencies and are employed in unidirectional airflow benches, air handlers, and as terminal air supply filters in cleanrooms.

Hepatic clearance Hepatic clearance is the volume of drug containing plasma that is cleared by the liver per unit time.

Heparin It is a sulphur containing polysaccharide, which stops blood from clotting by preventing the conversion of prothrombin to thrombin and by neutralizing thrombin.

Hepatic herbs Herbs that promotes the well-being of the liver and increases the secretion of bile.

Hepatitis Infection, which results in inflammation of the liver.

Hepatitis A A type of hepatitis, which is transmitted by fecal-oral contamination, primarily affects children and young adults, especially in environments where there is poor sanitation and overcrowding. This disease is caused by the hepatitis A virus, which is a single-stranded RNA virus.

Hepatitis B This form of hepatitis is caused by a double-stranded DNA virus (HBV) and the virus is transmitted by body fluids.

Hepatitis C About 90% of all cases of viral hepatitis can be traced to either HAV or HBV and the remaining 10% is believed to be caused by one and possibly several other types of viruses of which one of these is hepatitis C.

Hepatitis D The liver disease, which is caused by the hepatitis D virus in those individuals who were already infected with the hepatitis B virus.

Hepatitis E The liver disease, which is caused by the hepatitis E virus, usually, a subclinical, acute infection results, but, there is a high mortality in women those who are in their last trimester of pregnancy.

Hepatotoxin A toxin, which is destructive to parenchymal cells of the liver.

Herb The word herb, also referred as botanical, has several different meanings depending on the perspective like plant which does not produce wood or plant or part of a plant used for medicinal, taste or aromatic purposes or refers to the aerial parts or the above-ground parts of plants which may include the flower, leaf, and the stem of the plant, and occasionally fruits too.

Herbaceous Term that is applied to a nonwoody stem or a plant with minimal secondary growth.

Herbal infused oils A process of extraction in which the volatile oils of a plant substance are obtained by soaking the plant in a carrier oil for approximately two weeks and then straining the oil. The resulting oil is used therapeutically and may contain the plant's aromatic characteristic.

Herbal medicinal product Any medicinal product, exclusively containing as active ingredients one or more herbal substances or one or more herbal preparations, or one or more such herbal substances in combination with one or more such herbal preparations

Herbal medicine An approach to healing which uses plant or plant derived preparations to treat, prevent, or cure various health conditions and ailments.

Herbal preparations Preparations, which are obtained by subjecting herbal substances to treatments such as extraction, distillation, expression, fractionation, purification, concentration or fermentation. These include comminuted or powdered herbal substances, tinctures, extracts, essential oils, expressed juices and processed exudates.

Herbal substances All mainly whole, fragmented or cut plants, plant parts, algae, fungi, lichen in an unprocessed, usually dried form, but sometimes fresh. Certain exudates that have not been subjected to a specific treatment are also considered to be herbal substances. Herbal substances are precisely defined by the plant part used and the botanical name according to the binomial system (genus, species, variety and author).

Herbalism Using natural plants or plant-based substances to treat a range of diseases and to enhance the functioning of the body's systems.

Herbicide A pesticide that is used to control weeds.

Herd immunity The resistance of a population to infection and spread of an infectious organism because of the immunity of a high percentage of the population.

Heredity Transfer of genetic information from parent cells to offspring.

Hermaphrodite Having both male and female reproductive organs, capable of forming male and female gametes on the same individual.

Herpatic A remedy for skin eruptions, ringworm, etc.

Herpetic keratitis An inflammation in the cornea and conjunctiva of the eye that results from a herpes simplex virus infection.

Hesperetin A flavanone.

Hetero (prefix) Two or more kinds of things.

Heterobimetallic complex A metal complex, which have two different metal atoms.

Heterocarpy When two morphologically different kinds of fruit are produced in the one inflorescence, it is said to be heterocarpy.

Heterocysts Refers to specialized cells, which are produced by cyanobacteria that are the sites of nitrogen fixation.

Heteroduplex DNA A double-stranded stretch of DNA formed by two slightly different strands

which are not completely complementary.

Heterogamous Sexual reproduction where gametes are not identical in shape or size.

Heterogeneous nuclear RNA The RNA transcript of DNA made by RNA polymerase II, which is then processed to form mRNA.

Heterogeneous Said, when there are two or more kinds of ray systems within an individual.

Heterolactic fermenters Microorganisms, which ferment sugars to form lactate, and also other products such as ethanol and CO_2.

Heteroleptic Transition metal or main group compounds, which have more than one type of ligand.

Heterolysis The cleavage of a bond by the process heterolytic cleavage or heterolytic fission, so that both bonding electrons remain with one of the two fragments between which the bond is broken.

Heteromorphic Having two or more distinct forms.

Heterophyllous Producing two or more leaf morphologies during the life of a plant.

Heteroreceptor Receptor that regulates the synthesis and/or the release of mediators other than its own ligand.

Heterotrophic organisms Organisms, which are not able to synthesize cell components from carbon dioxide as sole carbon source.

Heterotrophs One of the two categories in which the microorganisms are classified on the basis of their carbon source. They use organic compounds such as carbohydrates, lipids, and hydrocarbons as a carbon and energy source.

Heterozygosity Presence of different alleles at one or more loci on homologous chromosomes.

Heterozygote An organism or cell that has two different alleles at corresponding loci on homologous chromosomes.

Hexon or hexamer Refers to a capsomer composed of six protomers.

Hexose A six carbon sugar, e.g. fructose, sucrose.

Hfr strain A bacterial strain, which donates its genes with high frequency to a recipient cell during conjugation because the F factor is included into the bacterial chromosome.

High oxygen diffusion environment A microbial environment, which is in close contact with air and through which oxygen can move at a rapid rate in comparison with the slow diffusion rate of oxygen through water.

Hildebrand parameter A parameter that measures the cohesion of a solvent.

Hilum The scar on a seed marking the place where it was attached to the seed stalk.

Hirsute Set with bristles or hairy or bushy.

Hispid With stiff hairs, spines, or bristles.

Histamine A compound with empirical formula $C_5H_9N_3$ which is found in tissues, released during allergic reactions and causes dilatation of capillaries, contraction of smooth muscle and stimulation of gastric acid secretion.

Histone A small basic protein, which has large amounts of lysine and arginine that is associated with eucaryotic DNA in chromatin.

Histoplasmosis A systemic fungal infection caused by *Histoplasma capsulatum*.

HIV therapies Offering a range of therapies that aim to treat the human immuno-deficiency virus, AIDS, or its' symptoms, these therapies are often used as complements to conventional approaches to HIV.

Hives Refers to an eruption of the skin.

Holdfast A structure produced by some bacteria and algae, which attaches the cell to a solid object.

Holistic A word targeted to the whole person-mind, body, and spirit. Holistic medicine not only considers physical health but also the emotional, spiritual, social, and mental well-being of the person.

Holoenzyme A complete enzyme that consists of the apoenzyme plus a cofactor.

Holozoic nutrition Nutrients, like bacteria, are acquired by phagocytosis and the subsequent formation of a food vacuole or phagosome is known as holozoic nutrition.

Homberg's salt Refers to boric acid, $B(OH)_3$.

Homeobox A short stretch of nucleotides whose base sequence is almost identical in all the genes which contains it, found in many organisms from fruit flies to human beings.

Homeopathy A medical system based on the belief that "like cures like", that illness can be cured by taking a minute dose of a substance that, if taken by a healthy person would produce symptoms like those being treated.

Homo (prefix) All alike, the same.

Homocellular Of plants, when an individual xylem ray has cells of a single kind.

Homogamous With flowers of only one kind with respect to their fertile organs in an inflorescence.

Homogeneous Of plants, when xylem rays within an individual hare of a single kind only.

Homolactic fermenters Refers to organisms, which ferment sugars almost completely to lactic acid.

Homoleptic Transition metal or compounds that have only one type of ligand are said to be homoleptic.

Homologous chromosome Chromosome that contains the same linear gene sequences as another, each derived from one parent.

Homologue A compound that belongs to a series of compounds differing from each other by a repeating unit, such as a methylene group, a peptide residue, etc.

Homology Refers to the similarity in DNA or protein sequences between individuals of the similar species or among different species.

Homolysis The cleavage of a bond by the process homolytic cleavage or homolytic fission, so that each of the molecular fragments between which the bond is broken retains one of the bonding electrons.

Homomorphic Superposable ligands are called homomorphic.

Honeydew An excretion from insects, such as aphids, mealy bugs, white flies, etc. that consists of modified plant sap.

Horizontal gene transfer Refers to the process in that the genes are transferred from one mature, independent organism to another.

Hormogonia Small motile fragments which are produced by fragmentation of filamentous cyanobacteria and used for asexual reproduction and dispersal.

Hormone A type of chemical messenger that occurs both in plants and animals, which acts to inhibit or excite metabolic activities. The site of production of hormone is distant from the site of biological activity.

Host A plant or animal that provides food for another organism.

Host vector (HV) system In transplantation of a gene, the guest gene is carried by a vector, which is a larger DNA molecule, such as a plasmid, or a virus into which that gene is genetically engineered and which then propagates in the host.

HSA (human serum albumin) The main protein constituent of human serum, which has no prosthetic group and is soluble in water and dilute salt solution, sometimes used in the treatment of shock, hypoproteinemia, and erythroblastosis fetalis.

Human gene therapy Therapy that involves insertion of normal DNA directly into cells to correct a genetic defect.

Human genome The full collection of genes required to produce a human being.

Human immunodeficiency virus (HIV) A lentivirus that belongs to the family Retroviridae,which is associated with the onset of AIDS.

Humectant A substance used to obtain a moistening effect.

Humoral (antibody-mediated) immunity Also known as antibody-mediated immunity, which is the type of immunity that results from the presence of soluble antibodies in blood and lymph.

Humus The organic matter present in the soil, formed by the decomposition of plant and animal remains, contains a large number of elements necessary for plant-growth. Its colloidal nature improves the texture of the soil and its water-retaining capacity.

Huntington's disease An adult-onset disease that is characterized by progressive mental and physical deterioration and it is caused by an inherited dominant gene mutation.

Hyaline Refers to thin, membranous, transparent or translucent texture.

Hyaluronic acid An organic acid which is the most effective natural skin moisturizer.

Hybrid An offspring of the fusion of gametes from genetically different parents and of different species.

Hybridization The process involved in the formation of hybrid.

Hybridoma A hybrid cell that results from the fusion of a specific antibody producing spleen cell with a myeloma cell. Produced hybrid cell shows the growth characteristics of the myeloma component and the antibody secreting characteristics of the spleen cell and will multiply to become a source of large quantities of pure, monoclonal antibody.

Hydathodes An epidermal structure that is specialized for secretion, or for exudation, of water.

Hydnocarpic acid A cyclopentenyl fatty acid.

Hydrastine An isoquinoline alkaloid.

Hydration Refers to the addition of water or the elements of water, (i.e. H and OH) to a molecular unit.

Hydric Characterized by an plentiful supply of water.

Hydrochloric acid A strong, corrosive inorganic acid, which is produced in the stomach to help digestion.

Hydrogen bond The hydrogen bond is a form of association between an electronegative atom and a hydrogen atom that is attached to a second, relatively electronegative atom.

Hydrogen bonding Strong type of intermolecular dipole-dipole attraction, which occurs between hydrogen and F, O or N.

Hydrogen peroxide It is a colorless, heavy, strongly oxidizing, unstable liquid used mainly in aqueous solutions as an antiseptic, bleaching agent, oxidizing agent, and laboratory reagent.

Hydrogenase Refers to an enzyme, dihydrogen acceptor oxidoreductase, which catalyzes the formation or oxidation of H_2.

Hydrogenosome A organelle like microbody that contains a unique electron transfer pathway in which hydrogenase transfers electrons to protons and molecular hydrogen is formed.

Hydrolase An enzyme, which catalyzes the hydrolysis of a substrate.

Hydrolysis A chemical reaction between water and organic compounds, particularly esters, ketones, and alcohols, which can lead to breakdown of some proteins.

Hydrolyzable tannins Including gallotannins and ellagitannins, complex esters of gallic acid with a carbohydrate (usually glucose), the ester linkages may be hydrolyzed by boiling with dilute hydrochloric acid, usually amorphous, hygroscopic, yellow-brown substances which dissolve in water to form colloidal rather than true solutions.

Hydrophilic With a strong affinity for water. Its opposite is hydrophobic.

Hydrophobic With a less affinity for water, non-wetting; water repelling.

Hydrophobic interaction The tendency of hydrocarbons or of lipophilic hydrocarbon-like groups in solutes, to form intermolecular aggregates in an aqueous medium, and analogous intramolecular interactions.

Hydrophyte Refers to aquatic plants living on or in water.

Hydroquinones A class of quinones, aromatic phenolic compounds in which two atoms of hydrogen are replaced by two hydroxy groups.

Hydrosol The water, which is obtained along with essential oil after plant materials are distilled. They are sometimes used in aromatherapy together with the essential oils and may be spritzed in the air and on the face and body.

Hydrotherapy Use of water as a medical treatment.

Hydroxyl group It is a functional group, which consists of an oxygen atom bonded to a hydrogen atom (:OH).

Hygienic Pertains to any equipment that by design, materials of construction, and operation provide for the maintenance of cleanliness, pyrogen free but not sterile, so that products formed by these systems will not adversely affect human or animal health.

Hygro (prefix) Water or moisture.

Hygroscopic A substance which readily attracts and retains water.

Hygroscopicity Refers to the affinity for absorbing water.

Hyoscyamine A tropane alkaloid.

Hypanthium An expansion of the receptacle of a flower, which forms a saucer-shaped, cup-shaped, or tubular structure, mostly like a calyx tube, bearing the perianth and stamens at or near its rim.

Hyperalimentation Administration of food through an intravenous tube in order to provide nutrition to a patient who cannot ingest food orally.

Hyperendemic disease A disease, which has a gradual increase in occurrence beyond the endemic level, but not at the epidemic level, in a given population.

Hyperglobulinemia (hypergammaglobulinemia) Term used to indicate high levels of antibody molecules in the blood of individuals those who are suffering from systemic inflammatory disease.

Hyperkeratosis Refers to the excessive scaliness of skin, scales of psoriasis represent a form of hyperkeratosis.

Hypermutation A rapid production of multiple mutations in a gene or genes through the activation of special mutator genes and the process may be deliberately used to maximize the possibility of creating desirable mutants.

Hyperpigmentation Production of increased amounts of melanin pigment in the skin that gives brown and black coloration.

Hypersensitivity Refers to the condition of increased immune sensitivity in which the body reacts to an antigen with an exaggerated immune response, which usually harms the individual. It is also termed as allergy.

Hypertonic Any solution having a high concentration of solute.

Hypertrophy Excessive growth due to increase in cell size.

Hypha Thread-like filaments, which form the mycelium (body) of a fungus.

Hypnosis Even though the condition resembles normal sleep, the brain wave patterns of hypnotized subjects are much closer to the patterns of deep relaxation. Also it is a process used to relax a patient, reduce resistance to therapy, facilitate memory, to address stopping smoking, eating less or to fight fears.

Hypnotic That tends to produce sleep.

Hypochlorite Weak, unstable salt of hypochlorous acid employed in aqueous solutions as a bleach, oxidizer, deodorant and disinfectant.

Hypocotyls Refers to the portion of an embryo or seedling that is between the cotyledons and the developing root tip.

Hypodermis Differentiated layer of cells below the epidermis.

Hypoferremia State of deficiency of iron in the blood.

Hypopigmentation Production of decreased amounts of melanin pigment in the skin leading to light colored or white areas.

Hypotheca Refers to the smaller half of a diatom frustule.

Hypothesis A tentative assumption or guess developed to explain a set of observations.

Hypotonic Any solution having a smaller osmotic pressure than that of the solution with it is being compared or a solution having a low concentration of solute.

Hypoxic With a low oxygen level.

Hypsochromic shift Shift of a spectral band to higher frequency or shorter wavelength upon substitution or change in medium. It is informally referred to as blue shift.

I

IAA Indole-acetic acid, a natural growth hormone that is found in plants.

ICH International conference on harmonisation.

ICSR Individual case safety report.

Ideal gas law PV=nrt, describes the relationship between pressure (P), temperature (T), volume (V), and moles of gas (n). It is not completely accurate, and becomes less accurate as conditions become less ideal.

Identity reaction A chemical reaction whose products are chemically identical with the reactants.

Idioblast Exactly, a unique cell, a clearly distinct, specialised and/or differentiated cell.

IgA Immunoglobulin A, class of immunoglobulins, which is present in dimeric form in many body secretions, (e.g. saliva, tears, and bronchial and intestinal secretions) and protects body surfaces. Also it is present in serum.

IgD Immunoglobulin D, class of immunoglobulins that is found on the surface of many B lymphocytes. It is thought to serve as an antigen receptor in the stimulation of antibody synthesis.

IgE Immunoglobulin E, class that binds to mast cells and basophils, and is responsible for type I or anaphylactic hypersensitivity reactions such as hay fever and asthma.

IgG Immunoglobulin G, the main immunoglobulin class in serum, which has functions such as neutralizing toxins, opsonizing bacteria, activating complement and crossing the placenta to protect the fetus and neonate.

IgM Immunoglobulin M, class of serum antibody which is first produced during an infection, large, pentameric molecule that is active in agglutinating pathogens and activating complement. On the surface of some B lymphocytes, the monomeric form is present.

Ileum The third and last section of the small intestine.

Imaging A medical diagnostic technique by which the organ images are obtained from the radiation emitted by radionuclides, which are introduced into organs, or from radiation absorbed by atomic nuclei within the organs.

Imbibition This takes place when a solvent enters a colloid between the free capillary spaces and the inter-micellar spaces. It causes the colloid to swell and ultimately to be dispersed.

Imbricate That has parts overlapping each other like roof tiles.

Immersed That grows under water.

Immune Exempt from infection by a given pathogen.

Immune complex The product of an antigen-antibody reaction that may also contain components of the complement system.

Immune response Formation of antibodies (humoral response) or particular types of cytotoxic lymphoid cells (cell-mediated response) on challenge with an antigen.

Immune system One of the eleven major body organ systems in vertebrates, which defends the internal environment against invading microorganisms and viruses and provides defense against the growth of cancer cells.

Immunity Refers to the overall general ability of a host to resist a particular disease or the condition of being immune..

Immunoelectrophoresis Separation of dissimilar antigen-antibody systems by diffusion in an agar gel, a separate precipitation band in the gel detects each system.

Immunoblotting The electrophoretic shifting of proteins from polyacrylamide gels to nitrocellulose sheets in order to demonstrate the presence of specific proteins through reaction with labeled antibodies.

Immunodeficiency A defect in the function of the immune system, which can be inherited or acquired, reversible or permanent.

Immunodiffusion A technique that involves the diffusion of antigen and/or antibody within a semisolid gel to create a precipitin reaction where they meet in proper proportions. Most often both the antibody and antigen diffuse through the gel, at times an antigen diffuses through a gel containing antibody.

Immunoelectrophoresis The electrophoretic partition of protein antigens, which is followed by diffusion and precipitation in gels using antibodies against the divided proteins.

Immunofluorescence A technique that is used to identify particular antigens microscopically in cells or tissues by the binding of a antibody conjugate that is fluorescent.

Immunogen A substance, which is capable of causing antibody formation.

Immunoglobulin (Ig) It is a member of a class of proteins, which functions as an antibody. According to the differences in their structure, the wide range of different specifities of antibodies are defined.

Immunology The branch of science, which deals with the immune system and many phenomena that are responsible for both acquired and innate immunity. It also includes the use of antibody-antigen reactions that comes under serology and immunochemistry.

Immunopathology Immunopathology is the study of diseases or conditions that results from immune reactions.

Immunoprecipitation A reaction that involves soluble antigens reacting with antibodies to form a large aggregate, which precipitates out of solution.

Immunoproteins Refers to all the proteins concerned with the immune system like antibodies, interferon and cytokines.

Immunotoxin A monoclonal antibody, which has been attached to a specific toxin or toxic agent and can kill particular target cells.

Imperfect flower A flower, which contains stamen and pistil organs required for pollination but lacking sepals or petals or both of these organs.

Impetigo Superficial cutaneous disease, which is most commonly seen in children, characterized by crusty lesions, generally located on the face, lesions typically have vesicles surrounded by a red border. It caused by *S. pyogenes* and also by *S. aureus*.

Imprinting A biochemical phenomenon that determines, which one of the pair of alleles, the mother's or the father's, will be active in that individual.

Impurity Any component that is present in the intermediate or active pharmaceutical ingredient, which is not the desired entity, which may be either process or product related.

Impurity profile A detailed description of the identified and unidentified impurities present in a usual batch of active pharmaceutical ingredient (API) that is produced by a specific controlled production process, which includes the identity or some qualitative analytical description, the range of each impurity observed, and type of each identified impurity. For every API, there should be an impurity profile describing the identified and unidentified impurities present in a typical batch.

In vitro Means, 'in glass', usually refers to any scientific studies performed on cells cultured in petri dishes that is contrasted to *in vivo*, which means 'in the living organism'.

Inactive ingredient Refers to any constituent other than an active ingredient.

Inactivation Process, which destroys the ability of a specific microbiological agent or eukaryotic cell to self-replicate.

Inclusion bodies Refers to the granules of organic or inorganic material, which is lying in the cytoplasmic matrix of bacteria.

Inclusion conjunctivitis An acute infectious disease, which happens throughout the world and is caused by *Chlamydia trachomatis* that infects the eye and causes inflammation and the occurrence of large inclusion bodies.

Incised Cut deeply, sharply and frequently irregularly.

Incontinence A condition, the inability to control the movement and passage of urine or bowel movements.

Incorporate To mix a material by mechanical action.

Incubatory carrier A person who is incubating a pathogen in large numbers but is not yet ill.

Incumbent Refers to the orientation of an embryo, with the cotyledons lying face to face and folded sideways so that the radicle lies against the face of one of the cotyledons.

Incurved Bent or curved upwards, inwards or adaxially.

Indehiscent Refers to fruits that do not open to release seeds, but whole fruit is shed from the plant, not opening to release the spores.

Index case The first disease case in an epidemic inside a given population.

Indicator organism An organism whose presence indicates the condition of a body or environment, the potential presence of pathogen Coliforms are used as indicators of fecal pollution.

Indigenous Refers to native, originating or occurring naturally in the place specified.

Indigenous species An indigenous species is one, which naturally grows within a particular part of the total species range and whose genetic material has adapted to that particular locality.

Indole alkaloids Alkaloids, which contain an indole ring and derived from phenylalanine or tryptophane.

Inducer A small molecule, which stimulates the synthesis of an inducible enzyme.

Inducible enzyme An enzyme whose level rises due to the presence of a small molecule, which stimulates its synthesis (see inducer).

Industrial ecology Ecological study of industrial societies with a major focus on material cycling, energy flow and the ecological impacts of such societies.

Inert Does not react chemically with other substances.

Infarct A necrotic tissue resulting due to the failure of local blood supply.

Infected Contaminated by means of extraneous biological agents and so capable of spreading infection.

Infection The invasion of a host by a microorganism following establishment and multiplication of the microorganism.

Infection thread It is a tubular structure, which is formed during the infection of a root by nitrogen-fixing bacteria. These bacteria enter the root by way of the infection thread and stimulate the formation of the root nodule.

Infectious Able to cause disease in a vulnerable host.

Infectious agent A biological organism that can cause disease in a vulnerable host.

Infectious disease Refers to any change from a state of health in which part or all of the host's body cannot carry out its normal functions due to the presence of an infectious agent.

Infectious disease cycle The cycle of events, which describes how an infectious organism grows, reproduces and is dispersed.

Infectious dose 50 (ID50) Refers to the dose or number of organisms, which will infect 50% of an experimental group of hosts within a particular time period.

Infectious mononucleosis An acute infectious disease of the lymphatic system, which is caused by the Epstein-Barr virus and characterized by fever, sore throat, lymph node and spleen swelling, and the proliferation of monocytes and abnormal lymphocytes.

Infectivity The state or quality of being infectious or communicable.

Infestation The presence of a huge number of insect organisms in an area, on the surface of a host or anything that might contact a host, or in the soil.

Infiltration The entry of air from a nearby room or from outside through wall and ceiling openings because of the difference in air pressure between the two areas.

Inflammation A localized protective response to tissue injury or destruction, which is characterized by pain, heat, swelling and redness in the injured area.

Inflorescence A group of flowers.

Influenza or flu A contagious disease that is caused by various strains of virus, characterized by fever, prostration, severe pains and progressive inflammation of the respiratory mucous membrane. This is caused by three strains of influenza virus, labeled types A, B and C, based on the antigens of their protein coats.

Informatics Refers to the study of the application of computer and statistical techniques to the management of information.

Infusion A tea made by pouring boiled water over plant material (usually dried flowers, fruit, leaves, and other parts, though fresh plant material may also be used), then allowed to steep.

Inhalation Movement of air from the external environment, through the airways, into the alveoli during breathing.

Injectable Able to be forced into the body through the surface of the skin and into a blood vessel.

Injection A preparation that is intended for parenteral administration and/or constituting or diluting a parenteral article prior to administration.

INN International non-proprietary name.

Inner bark In older trees, the living part of the bark, the phloem.

Inoculum Any stage of a pathogen, such as spores or virus particles, which can infect a host.

Inorganic Without carbon, generally used to indicate materials that are of mineral origin.

In-process control Also called as process control, checks performed during production to monitor and if required to adjust the process and/or to ensure that the intermediate or active pharmaceutical ingredient conforms to its specification.

Insecticide An herb or substance that kills insects.

Insectivorous Catching and feeding on insects.

Insertion A type of mutation in that a new DNA base is inserted into an existing sequence of DNA bases.

Insulin A hormone that is produced by the pancreas, which regulates the metabolism of glucose in the body.

Integration The incorporation of one DNA section into a second DNA molecule in order to form a new hybrid DNA.

Integrins They are a large and broadly distributed family of a/b heterodimers, cellular adhesion receptors, which mediate cell-cell and cell-substratum interactions.

Integrated pest management Pest control methods using a group of complementary approaches that includes natural predators, parasites, pest-resistant plant varieties, pesticides and other biological and environmental control practices.

Integumentary system System refers to the skin and its derivatives like, hair, nails, feathers, horns, antlers, and glands, which in multicellular animals protect against invading foreign microorganisms and prevent the loss or exchange of internal fluids.

Inteins Internal superseding sequences of precursor self-splicing proteins, which separate exteins and are removed during the formation of the final protein.

Interaction An effect, which is produced when two drugs are administered at the same time and the effectiveness of one or both of the drugs is either enhanced or diminished by the other.

Intercellular Lying between cells, as intercellular space in plant tissue.

Interfascicular cambium A lateral meristem that develops from tissues in the region between the vascular bundles, and, with the fascicular cambium that makes up the vascular cambium.

Interfascicular region Tissues between the vascular bundles.

Interference In biology, the overall influence of one plant or group of plants on another, and includes allelopathy or competition, or both of these processes.

Interferon Refers to a group of proteins released by the immune system, which inhibit the growth of an infection caused by viruses.

Interleukin Group of glycoproteins produced by the leukocytes in the immune system, which aid in the formation of lymphocytes.

Intermediate meristem Of a root apical meristem in that the cell files giving rise to dissimilar tissues trace to the initials at the apex, but the initials are not clonally distinct.

Intermolecular Descriptive of any process, which involves a transfer of atoms, groups, electrons, etc. or interactions between two or more molecular units.

Intermolecular forces Refers to forces between molecules.

Internal phloem Primary phloem, which is found adaxially or internally to the xylem in the stem, in

the leaf clear as a bicollateral vascular bundle.

Internode Refers to the portion of a stem between nodes.

Interpetiolar Refers to stipules that is between the petioles of two opposite leaves.

Interstitial fluid Fluid surrounding the cells in body tissues, which provides a path through which nutrients, gases and wastes can travel between the capillaries and the cells.

Interstitial lung disease A type of pneumonia not caused by infections, which can produce shortness of breath in patients having dermatomyositis, scleroderma or other forms of rheumatic disease. Also known as interstitial pneumonia or interstitial pneumonitis.

Intestinal flora The friendly bacteria, which are present in the intestines.

Intoxication A disease, which results from the entry of a specific toxin into the body of a host and the toxin can induce the disease in the absence of the toxin-producing organism.

Intra-arterial injection The drug is injected into a specific artery to achieve a high drug concentration in a specific tissue before drug distribution occurs throughout the body. Intra-arterial injection is used for diagnostic agents and occasionally for chemotherapy.

Intra-articular injection The drug is injected into a joint.

Intracellular Within a body cell or within the body cells.

Intradermal (intracutaneous) injection The drug is injected into the dermis, (i.e. the vascular region of the skin below the epidermis).

Intraepidermal lymphocytes T cells, which are found in the epidermis of the skin, which express the gamma delta T cell receptor.

Intramolecular Descriptive of any process, which involves a transfer of atoms, groups, electrons, etc. or interactions between different parts of the same molecular unit.

Intramolecular catalysis The acceleration of a chemical alteration at one site of a molecular entity through the participation of another functional group in the same molecular entity, without that group appearing to have undergone change in the reaction product.

Intramolecular forces Refers to forces within molecules.

Intramuscular injection The drug is injected deep into a skeletal muscle. The rate of absorption depends on the vascularity of the muscle site, the lipid solubility of the drug, and the formulation matrix.

Intranuclear inclusion body It is a structure found within cells infected with the cytomegalovirus.

Intrathecal injection The drug is injected into the spinal fluid.

Intravenous Substance injected into a vein.

Intravenous bolus injection The drug is injected directly into the bloodstream, distributes throughout the body, and acts rapidly. Any side effects, including an intense pharmacologic response, anaphylaxis, or overt toxicity, also occur rapidly.

Intravenous infusion The drug is given intravenously at a constant input rate. Constant rate intravenous infusion maintains a relatively constant plasma drug concentration.

Intrinsic activity It is the maximal stimulatory response, which is induced by a compound in relation to that of a given reference compound.

Intrinsic factors Factors such as moisture, pH and available nutrients, which influence microbial growth.

Intron A noncoding intervening series in a split or interrupted gene that codes for RNA, which is missing from the final RNA product.

Inulin A fructan, which acts as a storage polysaccharide and yields fructose on hydrolysis.

Invasive alien species Species, which were introduced outside their natural distribution area, and which exhibit fast growth, reproduction and dispersal to an extent that they are highly competitive to native species. They were destructive and difficult to control, mainly if the new ecosystem lacks the predators or pathogens of their own native range. The spread of this species threatens the environment, the economy, or society, including human health.

Invasiveness Refers to the ability of a microorganism to enter a host, grow and reproduce within the host, and spread all over its body.

Inversion A reversal in the order of genes on a chromosome segment.

Invertebrate An animal that have no internal skeleton.

Inverted micelle The reversible formation of association colloids from surfactants in non-polar solvents leads to aggregates, which is termed inverted micelles.

Investigational new drug (IND) application A document filed with the FDA prior to clinical trial of a new drug. It gives a full description of the new drug, where and how is manufactured, all QC information, etc. The IND is followed by new drug application (NDA).

Ion Removing or adding electrons to an atom produces an ion, also a charged object very similar to an atom.

Ion-dipole forces Intermolecular force, which exist between charged particles and partially charged molecules.

Ion channel Ion channels facilitate ions to flow quickly through membranes in a thermodynamically downhill direction after an electrical or chemical impulse. Their structures typically consist of 4-6 membrane-spanning domains and this number decides the size of the pore and thus the size of the ion to be transported.

Ion pair A pair of oppositely charged ions that are held together by Coulomb attraction without formation of a covalent bond. Practically, an ion pair behaves as one unit in determining conductivity, osmotic properties, etc.

Ion pumps Ion pumps facilitate ions to flow through membranes in a thermodynamically uphill direction by the use of an energy source like ATP or light. They consist of sugar-containing hetero-peptide assemblies that open and close upon the binding and subsequent hydrolysis of ATP, generally transporting more than one ion towards the outside or the inside of the membrane.

Ionic bonds Said when two oppositely charged atoms share not less than one pair of electrons but the electrons spend more time near one of the atoms than the other.

Ionization Generation of one or more ions.

Ionization energy Energy required to eliminate an electron from a specific atom.

Ionizes Said when a substance breaks into its ionic components.

Ionizing power A word to indicate the tendency of a particular solvent to promote ionization of an uncharged or, less often, charged solute. This word is used both in a kinetic and in a thermodynamic context.

Ionizing radiation Radiation of very short wavelength or high energy, which causes atoms to lose electrons or ionize.

Ionophore A compound that can carry specific ions through membranes of cells or organelles.

Ipso-attack Attachment of an entering group to a position in an aromatic compound, which is already carrying a substituent group, other than hydrogen and the entering group may displace that substituent group but may also itself be migrated to a different position in a subsequent step.

Iridoids It is a subclass of terpenoids, monoterpenoids with lactone substitutions, frequently in glycosidic form.

Iridology It is a diagnostic system that is based on the premise that every organ has a corresponding location within the iris of the eye that can serve as an indicator of the organ's health or disease.

Iron-responsive element A specific base sequence in certain messenger RNAs, which code for various proteins of iron metabolism that allows regulation at translational level by the iron-responsive protein.

Iron-responsive protein (IRP) A protein, which responds to the level of iron in the cell, and regulates the biosynthesis of proteins of iron metabolism, by binding to the iron-responsive element on messenger RNA.

Iron-sulfur cluster A component encompasses two or more iron atoms and bridging sulfide ligands in an iron-sulfur protein.

Iron-sulfur proteins Proteins in that the non-heme iron is coordinated with cysteine sulfur and also with inorganic sulfur.

Ischemia Deficiency of blood supply and so dioxygen to an organ or tissue owing to constriction of the blood vessels.

Isobifacial Refers to flattened structures, particularly leaves, having both surfaces structurally similar.

Isodesmic reaction A reaction in that the types of bonds, which are made in forming the products are the same as those which are broken in the reactants.

Isoelectronic Molecular entities are described as isoelectronic if they have the same number of valence electrons and the same structure.

Isoentropic A reaction series is said to be isoentropic if the individual reactions of the series have the same standard entropy of activation.

Isoenzyme Any of the multiple forms of an enzyme each of which possesses different characteristics kinetic properties, usually obtained by different combinations of the same two or more subunits.

Isoflavans Refers to the isomeric form of flavones with the most reduced structure of any isoflavonoids, which lack hydroxy or ketone groups.

Isoflavones Refers to a class of flavonoids in which the B ring of flavones is attached to the 3-position, instead of the 2-position.

Isoflavonoids Refer to a class of flavonoids in which the B ring of flavones is attached to the 3-position, instead of the 2-position and, which lack the 3-hydroxy group of flavonols.

Isolobal Word that compare molecular fragments with each other and with familiar species from organic chemistry. Two fragments are called as isolobal if the number, symmetry properties, approximate energy, and shape of the frontier orbitals and the number of electrons in them are similar.

Isomer Two compounds are said to be isomers of each other when they have the same number and kinds of atoms, but those atoms are arranged in different ways. Otherwise, one of several chemical species, which have the same stoichiometric molecular formula but different constitutional formulae or different stereochemical formulae and so potentially different physical and/or chemical properties.

Isomerase An enzyme that catalyzes the isomerization of a substrate.

Isonome method Technique of studying plant distribution in a particular area that is having clear variations in species composition.

Isopathy Treatment of a disease with the same disease agent.

Isosbestic point Indicates a set of absorption spectra, plotted on the same chart for a set of solutions in which the sum of the concentrations of two principal absorbing components, A and B, is constant and the curves of absorbance against wavelength for such a set of mixtures often all intersect at one or more points, called isosbestic points.

Isosteres Isosteres are molecules of similar size containing the same number of atoms and valence electrons.

Isothiocyanates They are esters of isothiocyanic acid, with a pungent smell and a sharp taste, which is derived from glucosinolates undergoing an enzymatic reaction through the enzyme myrosinase when plant tissue is crushed.

Isotonic solutions An isotonic solution is one that has the same osmotic pressure as body fluids. Solutions to be administered to patients should be isosmotic with body fluids. A hypotonic solution is one with a lower osmotic pressure than body fluids, whereas a hypertonic solution will have an osmotic pressure that is greater than body fluids.

Isotope effect The effect on the rate or equilibrium constant of two reactions, which differ only in the isotopic composition of one or more of their otherwise chemically identical components is referred isotope effect.

Isotope effect, kinetic The effect of isotopic substitution on a rate constant is known as a kinetic isotope effect.

Isotope effect, solvent A kinetic or equilibrium isotope effect that results from change in the isotopic composition of the solvent.

Isotope effect, steric A secondary isotope effect, which is attributed to the different vibrational amplitudes of isotopologues.

Isotope effect, thermodynamic The effect of isotopic substitution on an equilibrium constant is known as a thermodynamic isotope effect.

Isotope exchange A chemical reaction in that the reactant and product chemical species are chemically same but have dissimilar isotopic composition. In this reaction, the isotope distribution tends towards equilibrium as a result of transfers of isotopically different atoms or groups.

Isotopes Elements that have same number of protons but different numbers of neutrons, and so different masses.

Isotopic tracer Any stable or radioactive isotope that is used to label a metabolite by incorporating it in place of normally incorporated isotope. As a result it could be followed in the metabolic pathway in the living organism, e.g. C isotope is incorporated into CO_2 taken up by a plant to know the photosynthetic pathway in photosynthesis.

Isotopologue A molecular entity, which differs only in isotopic composition.

Isotopomer Isomers that have the same number of each isotopic atom but differs in their positions.

Isotropy The property of molecules and materials of having identical physical properties in all directions.

Isoquinoline alkaloids Refers to a group of alkaloids that are having structure based on isoquinoline nucleus and derived from amino acid tyrosine and phenylalanine, e.g. morphine.

Isotype A variant form of an immunoglobulin, which occurs in every normal individual of a particular species.

Isovitexin A glycoflavones.

IU International Unit. A measure of potency based on an accepted international standard.

J

J chain A polypeptide present in polymeric IgM and IgA that links the subunits together.

Jaccard coefficient (SJ) An association coefficient used in numerical taxonomy; it is the proportion of characters that match, excluding those that both organisms lack.

Jaculator A hardened and hook-like funicle that is conspicuous in the seeds of many Acanthaceae.

Jaundice A disease characterized by obstruction of bile, leading to yellowing of the skin, fluids, and tissues, by weakness, by constipation, and by loss of appetite.

Jejunum The second portion of the small intestine.

Jo-1 antibody A type of antibody molecule seen in the blood of patients with muscle inflammation due to polymyositis or dermatomyositis.

Jugate Juicy or fleshy.

Juvenile Refered to leaves, those on a young plant different in form from those on an adult, sometimes also occurring on sucker or reiterating shoots.

K

Kaempferol A common flavonol with a single hydroxyl group attached to the B ring, which occurs as a copigment in flowers and fruits.

Karma Refers to the basic concept that is common to Hinduism, Buddhism, and Jainism. The doctrine holds that one's state in this life is the result of physical and mental actions in past life and that present action can determine one's destiny in future life. Karma is a natural, impersonal law of moral cause and effect.

Karyotype A photomicrograph of an individual's chromosomes arranged in a standard format showing the number, size and shape of each chromosome type. It is used in low-resolution physical mapping to correlate gross chromosomal abnormalities with the characteristics of specific diseases.

Keratins Refer to insoluble protective or structural proteins consisting of parallel polypeptide chains in α-helical or β-conformation.

Ketose A simple monosaccharide having its carbonyl groups at other than a terminal position.

Kinase An enzyme that catalyzes phosphorylation of an acceptor molecule by adenosine triphosphate (ATP).

Keel The folded edge or ridge of any structure.

Kekule structure (for aromatic compounds) A representation of an aromatic molecular entity, (e.g. benzene), with fixed alternating single and double bonds, in which interactions between multiple bonds are assumed to be absent.

Kelvin The SI unit of temperature, degrees celsius plus 273.

Kelp Refers to the common name for any of the larger members of the order Laminariales of the brown algae.

Keratinocyte The most common type of cell in the epidermis, protective outer stratum corneum layer is made up of dead keratinocytes, which have become stuck together.

Keratitis Inflammation of the cornea of the eye.

Kernel Refers to endosperm, embryo, etc.

Kestose Refers to a frutosyl sucrose oligosaccharide, which may serve as intermediates in the biosynthesis of fructans.

Ketones Ketones have a general formula of $R - CO - R$ and, similar to aldehydes, they contain a carbonyl group $(C = O)$.

Kidney stones Crystallized deposits of excess wastes such as uric acid, calcium, and magnesium, which may form in the kidney.

kilocalorie The energy required to heat 1000 grams of water from 14.5 to 15.5 °C.

Kinesiology Refers to the study of muscles and their movement. Applied kinesiology is a system, which uses muscle testing procedures, in combination with standard methods of diagnosis, to gain information about a patient's overall state of health. Practitioners analyze muscle function, posture, gait and other structural factors in addition to lifestyle factors, which may be contributing to a health-related problem.

Kinetic control (of product composition) The term characterizes conditions, including reaction times, which lead to reaction products in a proportion governed by the relative rates of the parallel (forward) reactions in which the products are formed, rather than by the respective overall equilibrium constants.

Kinetic energy Refers to the energy an object has because of its mass and velocity.

Kinetic equivalence Two reaction schemes are kinetically equivalent, if they involve the same rate law.

Kinetic resolution Refers to the achievement of partial or complete resolution by virtue of unequal rates of reaction of the enantiomers in a racemate with a chiral agent.

Kinetoplast A special structure in the mitochondrion of kinetoplastid protozoa that contains the mitochondrial DNA.

Kingdoms Five broad taxonomic categories, Monera, Protista, Plantae, Fungi, Animalia, into which organisms are grouped, based on common characteristics.

King's yellow Refers to a native yellow arsenic(III) sulfide, As_2S_3.

Kirby-Bauer method A type of disk diffusion test to find out the susceptibility of a microorganism to chemotherapeutic agents.

Koch's postulates A set of rules for proving that a microorganism causes a particular disease.

Koplik's spots Lesions of the oral cavity caused by the measles (rubeola) virus, characterized by a bluish white speck in the center of each.

Korean hemorrhagic fever An acute infection caused by a virus, which produces varying degrees of hemorrhage, shock and at times death.

Kreb's cycle Biochemical cycle in cellular aerobic metabolism where acetyl CoA is combined with oxaloacetate to form citric acid; the resulting citric acid is converted into a number of other chemicals, eventually reforming oxaloacetate; NADH, some ATP, and $FADH_2$ are produced and carbon dioxide is released.

Kurrol's salt Refers to a potassium phosphate, $(KPO_3)_4$.

L

L (prefix) Laevo, handedness of isomers.

L-phenylalanine A non-protein amino acid from which isoquinoline alkaloids are derived through decarboxylation.

L-tryptophane Aromatic, neutral, hydrophobic, non-polar, amino acid.

L-tyrosine A non-protein amino acid, aromatic, polar, hydrophobic.

La/SS-B autoantibody A type of autoantibody that is seen in patients having certain forms of skin lupus like subacute cutaneous LE or neonatal LE and Sjögren's syndrome.

Labile Term used to describe either a relatively unstable and transient chemical species or a relatively stable but reactive species.

Laccase A copper-containing enzyme, 1,4-benzenediol oxidase, which are found in higher plants and microorganisms. They are multicopper oxidases of wide specificity that carry out one-electron oxidation of phenolic and related compounds, and reduce O_2 to water.

Lactagogue Agent that increases secretion of milk.

Lactate To secrete milk from the mammary glands.

Lactic acid fermentation Fermentation, which produces lactic acid as the sole or primary product.

Lactoferrin An iron-binding protein from milk, structure similar to the transferrins.

Lactones They are cyclic compounds with a 5-6 membered ring in which the chain is closed by ester formation between a carboxyl and a hydroxyl group in the same molecule.

Lacuna Refers to a gap or cavity.

Lacunate With air spaces or chambers in the midst of tissue.

Lag phase A period following the introduction of microorganisms or cells into fresh culture medium when there is no increase in cell numbers or mass during batch culture.

Lager Pertains to the process of aging beers to allow flavor development.

Lagoon A shallow lake or pond, especially one connected with a larger body of water; also an area of shallow salt water separated from the sea by sand dunes.

Lake An inland body of water, usually fresh water, formed by glaciers, river drainage, etc. larger than a pool or pond.

Lamina Any broad and flattened region of a plant or alga that allows for increased photosynthetic surface area.

Laminar airflow-clean work station A workstation in which the unidirectional airflow characteristics predominate throughout the entire air space with a minimum of turbulence to expose critical surfaces.

Laminar flow Non-turbulent fluid flow that is usually considered laminar if the Reynolds number is less than 2000 in a pipe.

Laminar flow hoods Worktables, which provide an enclosed sterile environment to protect solutions or media from contamination while they are prepared.

Lamination Lamination is separation of a tablet into two or more distinct layers. These problems are usually caused by entrapment of air during processing.

Lamella A thin, plate-like layer.

Lamellate Made up of lamina or thin plates.

Laminarin Main storage products of the golden-brown algae, which is a polymer of glucose.

Land farming The addition of waste material, such as a hydrocarbon waste, to the soil surface so that it will be degraded. The soil may be moistened or mixed to stimulate the desired degradation process.

Langelier index It is a measure of the degree of saturation of calcium carbonate in water, which is based on pH, alkalinity and hardness. If the Langelier index is negative, the water is acidic (pH value below 7). If the Langelier index is positive, calcium carbonate can precipitate out of solution to form scale (pH value above 7 or basic). The Langelier index will vary for cold water and for warm water.

Langerhans cell Cell that is found in the skin, which internalizes antigen and moves in the lymph to lymph nodes where it differentiates into a dendritic cell.

Large intestine It consists of the cecum, appendix, colon, and rectum, absorbs some nutrients and drugs, but mainly prepares feces for elimination.

Larva The immature form of insects that develop through the process of complete metamorphosis including egg, several larval stages, pupa, and adult.

Larynx A hollow structure at the beginning of the trachea.

Late mrna Messenger RNA that is produced later in a virus infection, which codes for proteins needed in capsid construction and virus release.

Latent heat The sum of heat needed to change a unit of substance, such as water, from a solid to a liquid without change in temperature or pressure.

Latent period The time between when a vector obtains a pathogen and when the vector becomes able to transmit the pathogen to a new host. Also, the time between infection of a host plant and production of inoculum by the infection.

Latent virus infections Refers to virus infections in which the virus quits reproducing and remains dormant for a period before becoming active again.

Lateral meristem A meristem of stem or root arranged parallel with the sides of the organ in which they occur.

Lateral roots Roots extending away from the main, taproot, root.

Laterocytic Refers to stomata, with three or more distinct subsidiary cells partially (not at the apex or base) surrounding the guard cells.

Latex vessel Term used for describing a simple or branched tube usually anastomosing with other similar tubes, derived from the enlargement and union of a chain of cells and containing latex in it.

Latex A viscous fluid exuded from the cut surfaces of the leaves and stems.

Laticifers A system of long multi-nucleate tubes in which latex is found.

Laughing gas Nitrous oxide, N_2O.

Lauric acid A saturated fatty acid.

Laxative An herb or substance that promotes or induces a mild and painless evacuation of the bowels. It is stronger than an aperient, but not purgative, cathartic, or drastic.

Layby application An application, usually of fertilizer or herbicide, after the crop is well established; especially, an application at the latest time in the season when it is still possible to pass through the field with a tractor.

Layered tablets Layered tablets are prepared by compressing a tablet granulation around a previously compressed granulation. The operation is repeated to produce multiple layers.

Le Chatlier's principle This principle states that a system at equilibrium will oppose any change in the equilibrium conditions.

Leach To dissolve something by the action of a moving liquid, e.g. high purity water leaches trace impurities from glass vessels.

Leaching Process used for the removal of mineral salts from the soil by percolating water.

Lead discovery It is the process of identifying active new chemical entities, which if required, by subsequent modification may be transformed into a clinically useful drug.

Lead generation Term applied to strategies developed to identify compounds which possess a desired but non-optimized biological activity.

Lead optimization Synthetic modification of a biologically active compound, modified to fulfill all stereoelectronic, physicochemical, pharmacokinetic and toxicologic required for clinical usefulness.

Leaf A lateral outgrowth from a stem that constitutes part of the foliage of a plant and functions primarily in food manufacture by photosynthesis. It consists of a flat lamina (blade) and a petiole (stalk). Many flowering plants have additionally a pair of small stipules near the base of the petiole.

Leaf area index The ratio between the total leaf surface area of a plant and the surface area of ground that is covered by the plant.

Leaf margin Refers to the outer edge of the leaf.

Leaf primordia Refers to young leaves, recently formed by the shoot apical meristem, located at the tip of a shoot.

Leaf veins They are vascular tissue in leaves, arranged in a net-like network (reticulate vennation) in dicots, and running parallel (parallel vennation) to each other in monocots.

Leaflet In a compound leaf, the individual blades are called leaflets.

Least nuclear motion, principle of The hypothesis that, for given reactants, the reactions involving the smallest change in nuclear positions will have the lowest energy of activation.

Leaving group An atom or group (charged or uncharged), which becomes detached from an atom in what is considered to be the residual or main part of the substrate in a specified reaction.

Lecithin A mixture of phospholipids, which is composed of fatty acids, glycerol, phosphorus, and choline or inositol, all living cell membranes are largely composed of lecithin.

Lectin complement pathway The lectin pathway for complement activation is triggered by the binding of a serum lectin to mannose-containing proteins or to carbohydrates on viruses or bacteria.

Lectins A group of hemagglutinating proteins (hemagglutinins), which are found primarily in plant seeds that bind specifically to the branching sugar molecules of glycoproteins and glycolipids on the surface of cells.

Leghemoglobin A monomeric hemoglobin, which is synthesised in the root nodules of leguminous plants that are host to nitrogen-fixing bacteria and has a high affinity for dioxygen and serves as an oxygen supply for the bacteria.

Legionnaires' disease A pulmonary form of legionellosis that results from infection with *Legionella pneumophila*.

Legume Refers to the fruit of Fabaceae, formed from one carpel and dehiscent along one or both sides, explosively so or not, or indehiscent, winged or not, splitting transversely or not.

Leishmanias Zooflagellates, members of the genus Leishma-

nia, which cause the disease leishmaniasis.

Leishmaniasis Refers to the disease caused by the protozoa called leishmanias.

Lenticel Corky spots on young bark that arise in relation to epidermal stomatas, through which gaseous exchange occur.

Lenticular Shaped like a double convex lens.

Lepromatous (progressive) leprosy A relentless, progressive form of leprosy in which large numbers of *Mycobacterium leprae* develop in skin cells, killing the skin cells and resulting in the loss of features.

Leprosy A severe disfiguring skin disease caused by *Mycobacterium leprae*.

Leptospira Genus of the family Treponemataceae, which are thin coiled organisms, flagellated at the extremities, one or both of which are bent back like a hook.

Lesion Refers to area of diseased or discolored tissue.

Lethal dose 50 (LD50) Refers to the dose that will kill 50% of an experimental group of hosts within a specified time period.

Leucoanthocyanins Proanthocyanidins.

Leukemia A progressive, malignant disease of blood-forming organs, that is marked by distorted proliferation and development of leukocytes and their precursors in the blood and bone marrow.

Leukocidin Refers to a microbial toxin that can damage or kill leukocytes.

Leukocyte Any colorless white blood cell that can be classified into granular and agranular lymphocytes.

Leukorrhea White viscous discharge from the vagina that results from inflammation of the mucous membrane.

Lewis acid A molecular entity, which is an electron-pair acceptor and therefore able to react with a Lewis base to form a Lewis adduct, by sharing the electron pair furnished by the Lewis base.

Lewis acidity The thermodynamic tendency of a substrate to act as a Lewis acid.

Lewis adduct Refers to the adduct formed between a Lewis acid and a Lewis base.

Lewis base A molecular entity, which is able to provide a pair of electrons and thus capable of coordination to a Lewis acid, thereby producing a Lewis adduct.

Lewis formula (electron dot or Lewis structure) Molecular structure in that the valency electrons are shown as dots so placed between the bonded atoms that one pair of dots represents two electrons or one (single) covalent bond.

Lewis structures A way of representing molecular structures based upon the valence electrons.

Lichen Refers to an organism composed of a fungus and either green algae or cyanobacteria in a symbiotic association.

Liebermann Burchard reagent Reagent used for the detection of the steroids and the triterpenes.

Liebig's law of the minimum Law states that living organisms and populations will grow until lack of a resource begins to limit further growth.

Ligaments Dense parallel bundles of connective tissues, which strengthen joints and hold the bones in place.

Ligand A molecule or ion that is bound to protein.

Ligase An enzyme that is used to catalyze the joining of single-stranded DNA segments.

Light reactions The photosynthetic process in which solar energy is harvested and transferred into the chemical bonds of ATP and it can occur only in light.

Lignan Colorless, crystalline, solid, dimeric compounds, which are derived from precursors related to those involved in the formation of lignin.

Lignin They are organic substances which act as binders for the cellulose fibers in wood and certain plants, and adds strength and stiffness to the cell walls, composed of a polymer of high carbon content but distinct from the carbonates and consists of C_6, C_3 units.

Lime Calcium oxide, CaO.

Lime-water A saturated aqueous solution of calcium hydroxide.

Limiting reagent The reactant, which will be exhausted first.

Limonene This is a monoterpene, which shows so much promise for cancer treatment, and also gives lemon scent to furniture polish and grease-cutting power to detergent.

Limonoids A type of triterpenoid (tetranortripterpenes), bitter compounds, pentacyclic, with a furan ring attached as a side chain.

Limulus amoebocyte lysate (LAL) A material obtained by rupturing the cellular components of the blood of a horseshoe crab (*Limulus poliphemus*). It coagulates in the presence of LPS (lipopoly-saccharides) and is a test used to quantitate bacterial endotoxins (pyrogens).

Line formula A two-dimensional representation of molecular entities in that the atoms are shown joined by lines representing single or multiple bonds, without any indication or implication concerning the spatial direction of bonds.

Line spectra Spectra generated by excited substances, consist of radiation with only specific wavelengths.

Linear Very narrow in relation to the length, and with the sides parallel.

Linear scleroderma A form of localized scleroderma, which takes the shape of a line or streak of abnormally hard or tight skin on an arm or leg, the body, or scalp. Internal organs such as the kidney, lungs and bowels are not affected by scleroderma changes.

Line-shape analysis This method is most often used in nuclear magnetic resonance spectroscopy that determines the rate constants for a chemical exchange from the shapes of spectroscopic lines of dynamic processes.

Liniment Extract of a plant or drug added to either alcohol or vinegar and applied topically to employ the therapeutic benefits.

Linkage The proximity of two or more markers, (e.g. genes) on a chromosome; the closer together the markers are, the lower the probability that they will be separated during DNA repair or replication processes, and hence the greater the probability that they will be inherited together.

Linnaean species A true origin of a species, in which many varieties have been included.

Lip Refers to a large projecting lobe of a corolla.

Lipase Refers to an enzyme which breaks down a true fat into its component fatty acid(s) and glycerol.

Lipid peroxidation Lipids, phospholipids in cell membranes and fatty acids in the bloodstream, are subject to attack by free radicals, which damage them by oxidation and this process is called lipid peroxidation.

Lipids Hydrophobic biological compounds (fats and fat-like materials) that are insoluble in water, but soluble in nonpolar solvents such as benzene, chloroform, and ether. The major components in most lipids are fatty acids.

Lipophilic Fat-loving, molecular entities (or parts of molecular entities) having a tendency to dissolve in fat-like, (e.g. hydrocarbon) solvents.

Lipophilicity Represents the affinity of a molecule or a moiety for a lipophilic environment.

Lipopolysaccharide A molecule containing both lipid and polysaccharide, which is important in the outer membrane of the gram-negative cell wall.

Lipoprotein A conjugated protein containing a lipid, prosthetic group.

Liposome An artificial phospholipid vesicle, useful for the enclosure of macromolecules such as nucleic acids or, after loading with an appropriate drug. It may be used therapeutically to achieve slow release of the drug into circulation.

Lipoxygenase A non-heme iron enzyme that catalyzes the insertion of O_2 into polyunsaturated fatty acids to form hydroperoxy derivatives.

Listeriosis A sporadic disease of animals and humans, particularly those who are immunocompromised or pregnant, caused by the bacterium *Listeria monocytogenes*.

Lithotriptic Causing the dissolution or destruction of stones in the bladder or kidneys.

Lithotroph Refers to an organism that uses reduced inorganic compounds as its electron source.

Loam Sand that have even proportions of sand, silt (mineral particle) and clay.

Lobed Refers to the apex of any laminar structure, e.g. petal, leaf blade, divided more than 25% the length of the structure.

Lobulate Divided into small lobes.

Localize Determination of the original position (locus) of a gene or other marker on a chromosome.

Localized scleroderma Localized scleroderma refers to a condition in which scleroderma produces hardening of the skin but does not attack the vital internal organs such as the kidney, lungs and bowels.

Location Where the symptom is experienced and location is one of the parts of a complete symptom.

Lone (electron) pair Two paired electrons localized in the valence shell on a single atom. Lone pairs are designated with two dots.

Long-day plant Refers to a plant that requires more than 12 hours of daylight before flowering will occur.

Long-day Refers to a photoperiodic response, where long periods of light alternating with short periods of dark are needed for flowering to occur.

Loop of Henle A U-shaped loop between the proximal and distal tubules in the kidney.

Lophotrichous A cell with a cluster of flagella at one or both ends.

Lotion It is a low to medium-viscosity medicated or non-medicated topical preparation intended for application to unbroken skin.

Low oxygen diffusion environment Refers to an aquatic environment in which microorganisms are surrounded by deep water layers that limit oxygen diffusion to the cell surface. In contrast, microorganisms in thin water films have good oxygen transfer from air to the cell surface.

Lower flammability level (LFL) The minimum concentration of vapor in air at which propagation of flame will occur in the presence of an ignition source, also, sometimes referred to as LEL or lower explosive limit.

Lower plant A plant without a vascular system.

LPS-binding protein A special plasma protein that binds bacterial lipopolysaccharides and then attaches to receptors on monocytes, macrophages, and other cells, which triggers the release of IL-1 and other cytokines that stimulate the development of fever and additional endotoxin effects.

Lubricants Lubricants reduce the friction that occurs between the walls of the tablet and the walls of the die cavity when the tablet is ejected. Talc, magnesium stearate, and calcium stearate are commonly used.

Lumen A cavity enclosed by a cell wall such as the central space of xylem vessel.

Lungs Sac-like structures of varying complexity where blood and air exchange oxygen and carbon dioxide, connected to the outside by a series of tubes and a small opening.

Lupinine A quinolizidine alkaloid.

Lupus A Latin word commonly used to refer to the autoimmune disease, lupus erythematosus.

Lupus band test It is a special microscopic examination of a skin biopsy specimen to determine if antibody or complement molecules are bound to the skin. This can be indicative of lupus erythematosus and can be performed on biopsies of lupus skin lesions (lesional lupus band test). It can also be performed on biopsies of normal, non-involved skin of lupus patients (non-lesional lupus band test).

Lupus erythematosus (LE) An autoimmune disease, which can attack virtually any organ in the body, including the skin. LE is extremely heterogeneous, which can cause a totally different set of problems from one patient to the next.

Lupus profundus A form of lupus skin disease in which knots form in the fatty layer of the skin, also known as lupus panniculitis.

Lupus rash A common term used for lupus skin disease.

Lutein Refers to a powerful antioxidant and one of two carotenoids, yellow pigments, found in the eye. These are believed to filter out harmful blue light and protect against age-related macular degeneration, the leading cause of blindness in people over 65.

Luteinizing hormone (LH) A hormone secreted by the anterior pituitary gland that stimulates the secretion of testosterone in men and estrogen in women.

Luteolin Hydroxylated flavone derivative, which is common in leaves and flowers.

Luteone An isoflavone.

LVP Large volume parenteral.

Lyases Refer to enzymes which breakdown complex molecules to simpler ones, without hydrolysis.

Lyate ion The anion produced by hydron removal from a solvent molecule, e.g. the hydroxide ion is the lyate ion of water.

Lycopene The pigment that gives tomatoes their red color and also makes grapefruit and watermelon pink.

Lymph node A small secondary lymphoid organ that contains lymphocytes, macrophages, and dendritic cells. It serves as a site for filtration and removal of foreign antigens and the activation and proliferation of lymphocytes.

Lymphatic system A network of glands and vessels that drain interstitial fluid from body tissues and return it to the circulatory system.

Lyophilizer A freeze dryer.

Lyophilization Also known as freeze drying, stabilizing wet substances by freezing them, then evaporating the resulting ice, to leave a substantially dry, porous residue which has the same size and shape of the original frozen mass.

Lymphocyte A type of white blood cell accounting for 20–25% of the white cells in humans, mostly non-phagocytic and actively mobile and is continuously made in the bone marrow. It is the immediate precursor of all antibody-forming cells.

Lymphokine A biologically active glycoprotein secreted by activated lymphocytes, especially sensitized T cells that act as an intercellular mediator of the immune response and transmit growth, differentiation, and behavioral signals.

Lysate A product of lysis that is the disintegration or dissolution of the cell walls.

Lysigenous Cavities in plants, formed by the dissolution of cells.

Lysine A basic amino acid obtained from many proteins by hydrolysis.

Lysis The dissolution or destruction of red blood cells, bacteria, or other antigens by a specific lysin, or by the action of detergents, therefore allowing the cell contents to escape.

Lysogens Bacteria, which are carrying a viral prophage and have the potential of producing bacteriophages under proper conditions.

Lysogeny The state in which a phage genome remains within the bacterial host cell after infection and reproduces along with it rather than taking control of the host and destroying it.

Lysosome It is a membrane-surrounded organelle in the cytoplasm of eukaryotic cells, contains many hydrolytic enzymes.

Lysozyme A substance present in some plants which has the capacity to kill bacteria.

Lytic cycle A virus life cycle, which results in the lysis of the host cell.

M

M cell Specialized cell of the intestinal mucosa and other sites, like the urogenital tract, which delivers the antigen from the apical face of the cell to lymphocytes clustered within the pocket in its basolateral face.

Maceration A process of softening tissues by soaking in liquid, a method of extraction.

Macro (prefix) Large, frequently used as an alternate for mega.

Macroalgae Large, macroscopic algae, seaweeds.

Macrolide antibiotic An antibiotic containing a macrolide (a large lactone ring with multiple keto and hydroxyl groups, linked to one or more sugars) ring.

Macromolecule A large molecule, which is a polymer of smaller units joined together (or) molecules whose molecular weights are greater than about 5,000 Daltons.

Macromolecule vaccine A vaccine, which is made of specific, purified macromolecules that are derived from pathogenic microorganisms.

Macronucleus The larger of the two nuclei in ciliate protozoa, normally polyploid and directs the routine activities of the cell.

Macronutrient Essential element, said of any element, which is required by the plant in relatively large amounts for its normal growth. Examples, carbon, hydrogen, oxygen, nitrogen, phosphorus, potassium, sulphur, magnesium, calcium and iron.

Macroparticle Particle with an equivalent diameter greater than 5 µm.

Macrophage The name for a large mononuclear phagocytic cell, present in blood, lymph, and other tissues, derived from monocytes. They phagocytose and destroy pathogens, some macrophages also activate B cells and T cells.

Macroreticular resin An ion exchange resin with a reticular porous matrix, which makes it effective for removing colloids and bacteria from process streams, as well as dissolved anions, useful for preventing colloidal and organic fouling of mixed-bed resins and premature clogging of final filters.

Macroscopic Items that are large enough to be observed by the naked eye.

Macrospore Megaspore.

Macrothallus Large, conspicuous phase of organisms, life history.

Maduromycosis Refers to a subcutaneous fungal infection caused by *Madurella mycetoma*, also termed as eumycotic mycetoma.

Madurose The sugar derivative 3-O-methyl-D-galactose that is characteristic of several actinomycete genera, which are collectively called maduromycetes.

Maesaquinone A benzoquinone.

Magnetic equivalence Nuclei having the same resonance frequency in nuclear magnetic resonance spectroscopy and also identical spin-spin interactions with the nuclei of a neighbouring group are magnetically equivalent. The spin-spin interaction between magnetically equivalent nuclei does not appear, and thus has no effect on the multiplicity of the respective NMR signals. Magnetically equivalent nuclei are also chemically equivalent, but the reverse is not necessarily true.

Magnetic resonance imaging (MRI) The visualization of the distribution of nuclear spins in a body by using a magnetic field gradient (NMR imaging).

Magnetic therapy Magnetic field therapy or bio-magnetic therapy involves the use of magnets, magnetic devices or magnetic fields inorder to treat a variety of physical and emotional conditions, including circulatory problems, certain forms of arthritis, chronic pain, sleep disorders, and stress.

Magnetosomes Magnetite particles in magnetotactic bacteria, which are tiny magnets and allow the bacteria to orient themselves in magnetic fields.

Magnetotactic Able to orient in a magnetic field.

Maintenance energy The energy a cell requires just to maintain itself or remain alive and functioning properly, which does not include the energy needed for either growth or reproduction.

Major histocompatibility complex (MHC) A large set of cell surface molecules in each individual, which is encoded by a family of genes, that serves as a unique biochemical marker of individual identity. It can trigger T cell responses, which may lead to rejection of transplanted tis-

sues and organs. These MHC molecules are also involved in the regulation of the immune response and the interactions between immune cells.

Makeup air Refers to the external air introduced to the air handling system for ventilation and pressurization.

Malar erythema Refers to redness over the cheeks of the face seen in systemic lupus patients.

Malaria A serious infectious illness that is caused by the parasitic protozoan Plasmodium, characterized by bouts of high chills and fever that occur at regular intervals.

Malegametophyte Refers to a plant body or cell lineage that is formed by vegetative growth of the microspore.

Malt Grain soaked in water to soften it, induce germination, activate its enzymes and this malt is then used in brewing and distilling.

Maltase It is an enzyme that breaks maltose into its component glucose molecules.

Mangiferin Xanthones.

Mannitol A hexitol that is formed by reduction of mannose or fructose, occurs in gum exudates.

Mannose Refers to a hexose sugar, an isomer of sucrose.

Mannuronic acid A type of uronic acid which occurs in seaweed gum alginic acid.

Mantra In Hinduism and Buddhism, mystic word used in ritual and meditation, believed to have power to bring into being the reality it represents. Use of these mantras usually requires initiation by a guru, or spiritual teacher.

Manufacture All operations of receipt of materials, production, packaging, repackaging, labelling, relabelling, quality control, release, storage and distribution of APIs and the related controls.

Manufacturer Refers to the party responsible for the quality of the drug product.

Manufacturing process All manufacturing and storage steps in the creation of the finished product from the weighing of components through the storing, packaging, and labeling of the finished product, including, but not limited to, mixing, granulating, milling, molding, formulating, lyophilizing, tableting, encapsulating, coating, sterilizing, and filling.

Manure Refers to the excreta of animals which is usually mixed with other material especially straw and used to improve soil fertility by adding it to soil.

Marburg viral hemorrhagic fever An acute infection caused by a virus, which produces varying degrees of hemorrhage, shock, and sometimes death.

Markers Chemically defined constituents of a herbal drug which are of interest for control purposes, independent whether they have any therapeutic activity or not. Markers may serve to calculate the quantity of herbal drug or preparation in the finished product if that marker has been quantitatively determined in the herbal drug or preparation when the starting materials were tested.

Marketing authorisation A licence, which is issued by a medicine agency approving the product for market based on a determination by the medicines agency that a pharmaceutical product meets the requirements of quality, safety and efficacy for human use in therapeutic treatment.

Mash Refers to the soluble materials released from germinated grains and prepared as a microbial growth medium.

Mashing The process in which cereals are mixed with water and incubated in order to degrade their complex carbohydrates (e.g. starch) to more readily usable forms such as simple sugars.

Mass number The number of protons and neutrons in an atom.

Massage therapy This is a general term for a range of therapeutic approaches that involves the practice of kneading or otherwise manipulating a person's muscles and soft tissue.

Mast cell A bone marrow-derived cell that is present in a variety of tissues that resemble peripheral blood-borne basophils and contain an Fc receptor for IgE, undergo IgE-mediated degranulation.

Materia medica In Latin materials of medicine, a reference that lists the curative indications and therapeutic actions of medicines.

Material A general term used to denote raw materials (starting materials, reagents, process aids, solvents), intermediates, APIs (active pharmaceutical ingredients) and packaging and labelling materials.

Matrix isolation A term that refers to the isolation of a reactive or unstable species by dilution in an inert matrix (argon, nitrogen, etc.) usually condensed on a window or in an optical cell at low temperature, inorder to preserve its structure for identification by spectroscopic or other means.

Matter Anything that has mass and occupies space.

Maturating Refers to an agent that promotes the maturing or bringing to a head of boils, carbuncles, etc.

Maximum working pressure Refers to the pressure at which the system is capable of operating for a sustained period.

Mayer's reagent Used in detection of alkaloids.

Mean growth rate constant (k) The rate of microbial population growth expressed in terms of the number of generations per unit time.

Mean kinetic temperature (MKT) The single calculated temperature at which the degradation of an article would be equivalent to the actual degradation, which results from actual temperature fluctuations during the storage period.

Mean residence time Mean residence time (MRT) is the average time for the drug molecules to reside in the body. MRT is also known as the mean transit time.

Measles A highly contagious skin disease, which is endemic throughout the world, caused by a morbilli virus in the family Paramyxoviridae that enters the body through the respiratory tract or through the conjunctiva.

Mechanical completion The point in a project at which all equipments and materials have been installed, but not started-up.

Mechanism A detailed description of the process leading from the reactants to the products of a reaction, including a characterization as complete as possible of the composition, structure, energy and other properties of reaction intermediates, products and transition states.

Mechanism-based inhibition Irreversible inhibition of an enzyme due to its catalysis of the reaction of an artificial substrate.

Media preparation The act of preparing nutrient media for cell/tissue culture or fermentation.

Median The median is the midmost value of a data distribution. When all the values are arranged in increasing (or decreasing) order, the median is the middle value for an odd number of observations. For an even number of observations, the median is the arithmetic mean of the two middle values. For a normal distribution, median equals mean.

Medical devices Any health care product, which does not achieve its principal intended purposes by chemical action in or on the body or by being metabolized. The term devices also include components, parts, or accessories of medical devices, diagnostic aids such as reagents, antibiotic sensitivity disks, and test kits for in vitro diagnosis of diseases and other conditions.

Medical mycology The discipline that deals with the fungi, which cause human disease.

Medicinal chemistry This is a chemistry-based discipline that involves aspects of biological, medical and pharmaceutical sciences, concerned with the invention, discovery, design, identification and preparation of biologically active compounds, the study of their metabolism, the interpretation of their mode of action at the molecular level and the construction of structure-activity relationships.

Medicinal plant Plants used by humans for therapeutic purposes.

Medicinal product Any substance or combination of substances presented for treating or preventing disease in human beings or animals, or, any substance or combination of substances that may be administered to human beings or animals with a view to making a medical diagnosis or to restoring, correcting or modifying physiological functions in human beings or in animals is likewise considered a medicinal product.

Meditation Discipline in which the mind is focused on a single point of reference.

Medium Refers to nutritive substance on or in which tissues or cultures of microorganisms may be grown.

Medulla A term referring to the central portion of certain organs. In plants, pith, a medullary bundle is a vascular bundle traversing the pith.

Medulla oblongata Refers to the region of the brain that, makes up the hindbrain, controls heart rate, constriction and dilation of blood vessels, respiration, and digestion.

Medullary ray A sheet of parenchyma that is running radially through the vascular tissue of a stem or root, which are concerned with food storage and lateral conduction of food materials water, etc. They may be primary or sec-

ondary, i.e. produced from the cambium when they are called vascular rays.

Megabase (Mb) Unit of length for DNA fragments equal to 1 million nucleotides and roughly equal to 1 Centimorgan (cM).

Megaphyll A large leaf, a leaf of any size whose vascular supply leaves one or more gaps as it departs from the stem vascular tissue.

Megasporangium Refers to a sporangium producing megaspores.

Meiosis Refers to the process of two consecutive cell divisions in the diploid progenitors of sex cells. It results in four rather than two daughter cells, each with a haploid set of chromosomes.

Melanin A pigment that gives the skin color and protects the underlying layers against damage by ultraviolet light, produced by melanocytes in the inner layer of the epidermis.

Melanocyte The type of cell in the epidermis that produces melanin pigment which gives normal skin its brown or tanned tone.

Melanoma A cancer, which begins in skin cells called melanocytes and spreads to internal organs.

Melatonin It is a hormone produced by the pineal gland in the brain and released mainly at night in the absence of light on the retina. Also it egulates the onset and timing of sleep and seasonal changes in the body such as winter weight gain. The levels of melatonin decline with age.

Membrane A barrier, usually thin polymer films, which only permits the passage of particles of a certain size or special nature, permeable to water and other fluids: 1. Microporous membrane filters have measurable pore structures that physically remove particles or microorganisms larger than pore size. 2. Ultrafiltration membranes (sometimes called molecular sieves) also remove molecules larger than a specified molecular weight. 3. Reverse osmosis membranes are permeable to water molecules and very little else, rejecting even dissolved ions and endotoxins in water.

Membrane-disrupting exotoxin A type of exotoxin, which lyses host cells by disrupting the integrity of the plasma membrane.

Membrane filter technique Use of a thin porous filter made from cellulose acetate or some other polymers to collect microorganisms from water, air, and food.

Membranous Having a thin, soft, pliable texture.

Memory B cell A lymphocyte, which is capable of initiating the antibody-mediated immune response upon detection of a specific antigen molecule for which it is genetically programmed. It circulates freely in the blood and lymph and may live for years.

Meniscoid Merging together or blending.

Meningitis A disease condition, which refers to inflammation of the brain or spinal cord meninges (membranes). It can be divided into bacterial (septic) meningitis (caused by bacteria) and aseptic meningitis syndrome (caused by nonbacterial sources).

Menkes' disease A sex-linked inherited disorder that causes defective gastrointestinal absorption of copper and resulting in copper deficiency early in infancy.

Menstrual cycle The recurring secretion of hormones and associated uterine tissue changes, characteristically 28 days in length.

Menthol An alcohol, which occurs in mint oils.

Mericarp One of the two carpels, which resembles achenes and forms the schizocarp of an umbelliferous plant.

Meristem Refers to group of undifferentiated cells from which new tissues are produced. The growing point or area of rapidly dividing cells at the tip of a stem, root, or branch

Meristem culture Used for describing the culture of excised meristems on suitable nutrient media under aseptic conditions (shoot tip culture).

Meristematic tissue Embryonic tissue located at the tips of stems and roots and occasionally along with their entire length; can divide to produce new cells.

Mescaline A protoalkaloid.

Mesenter Epithelial cells that support the digestive organs.

Mesocarp The fleshy middle portion of the wall or pericarp of a succulent fruit.

Meso-compound A term for the achiral member(s) of a set of diastereoisomers that also includes one or more chiral members.

Mesolytic cleavage Cleavage of a bond in a radical ion whereby a radical and an ion are formed. The term also reflects the mechanistic duality of the process that can be viewed as homolytic or heterolytic depending on how the electrons are attributed to the fragments.

Mesomeric effect The effect, on reaction rates, ionization equilibria, etc. attributed to a substituent due to overlap of its p or pi orbitals with the p or pi orbitals of the rest of the molecular entity.

Mesomerism The term is particularly associated with the picture of pi electrons as less localized in an actual molecule than in a Lewis formula.

Mesophase Refers to the phase of a liquid crystalline compound between the crystalline and the isotropic liquid phase.

Mesophile A microorganism with a growth optimum around 20 to 45°C, a minimum of 15 to 20°C, and a maximum about 45°C or lower.

Mesophyll Refers to the photosynthetic tissue in the leaf in particular (blade of a leaf), meaning middle of the leaf.

Mesophytic leaves The leaves of plants that grow under moderately humid conditions with plentiful soil and water.

Messenger RNA (mRNA) Single-stranded RNA that is synthesized from a DNA template during transcription that binds to ribosomes and directs the synthesis of protein.

Metabolic channeling Refers to the localization of metabolites and enzymes in different parts of a cell.

Metabolic control engineering Modification of the controls for biosynthetic pathways without altering the pathways themselves to improve process efficiency.

Metabolic pathway A series of individual chemical reactions in a living system, which combine to perform one or more important functions.

Metabolic pathway engineering (MPE) The use of molecular techniques to improve the efficiency of pathways, which synthesize specific products.

Metabolism The entire physical and chemical processes involved in the maintenance and reproduction of life in which nutrients are broken down to generate energy and to give simpler molecules (catabolism) which by themselves may be used to form more complex molecules (anabolism).

Metabolite Refers to any intermediate or product resulting from metabolism (or) any of the various organic compounds produced by metabolism.

Metalloenzyme An enzyme that, in the active state, contains one or more metal ions that are essential for its biological function.

Metallo-immunoassay Refers to a technique in which antigen-antibody recognition is used, with attachment of a metal ion or metal complex to the antibody. The specific absorption or (radioactive) emission of the metal is then used as a probe for the location of the recognition sites.

Metallothionein A small, cysteine-rich protein, which binds heavy metal ions, such as zinc, cadmium and copper in the form of clusters.

Metaphase Refers to a stage in mitosis or meiosis during which the chromosomes are aligned along the equatorial plane of the cell.

Metastases Plural of metastasis.

Metastasis In cancer, it is the appearance of neoplasms in parts of the body remote from the seat of the primary tumor. It also applies to the transportation of bacteria from one part of the body to another through the bloodstreams, hematogenous metastasis, or through lymph channels, lymphogenous metastasis.

Metathesis A bimolecular process formally that involves the exchange of a bond (or bonds) between similar interacting chemical species so that the bonding affiliations in the products are identical (or closely similar) to those in the reactants.

Metaxylem Refers to later formed primary xylem differentiating from the procambium, the tracheary elements having more or less continuously thickened walls with pits.

Methane mono-oxygenase A metalloenzyme, which converts methane and dioxygen to methanol using NADH as co-substrate. Two types are identified, one containing a dinuclear oxo-bridged iron center and the other is a copper protein.

Methanogens Strictly anaerobic archaea, which is able to use a variety of substrates, (e.g. dihydrogen, formate, methanol, methylamine, carbon monoxide or acetate) as electron donors for the reduction of carbon dioxide to methane.

Methods validation Setting up, through documented evidence, a high degree of assurance, which an analytical method will consistently yield results that accurately reflect the quality characteristics of the product tested.

Methoxy group Refers to a functional group consisting of an oxygen atom attached to a methyl group (:OCH_3).

Methyl cellulose A common viscosity-increasing agent, inversely soluble with temperature used in various preparations.

Methyl glucosinolates Refer to a class of aliphatic, straight chain glucosinolates.

Methyl group Refers to a functional group consisting of a carbon atom with three hydrogen atoms attached (:CH_3).

Methylazoxymethanol Refers to the toxic aglycone of cycasin and macrozamin.

Methylene blue 3,9-bisdimethyl-aminophenazothionium chloride trihydrate, $C_{16}H_{18}N_3SCl \cdot 3H_2O$, a thiazine dye and redox indicator.

Methylflavones Refer to derivatives of chalcones.

Me-too drug A me-too drug is a compound, which is structurally very similar to already known drugs, with only minor pharmacological differences.

Mevalonic acid A carboxylic acid precursor of sterols, terpenes and other isoprenoids.

Micellar catalysis The acceleration of a chemical reaction in solution by means of adding a surfactant at a concentration higher than its critical micelle concentration so that the reaction can proceed in the environment of surfactant aggregates (micelles).

Micelle Surfactants in solution are often association colloids, i.e. they tend to form aggregates of colloidal dimensions, which exist in equilibrium with the molecules or ions from which they are formed and these aggregates are termed micelles.

Microaerophile A microorganism, which requires low levels of oxygen for growth, around 2 to 10%, but is damaged by normal atmospheric oxygen levels.

Microarray technology Refers to the profiling of gene expression by measuring binding of RNA from growing cells to an array of function-specific oligonucleotides attached to an inert surface.

Microbe A microscopic one-celled organism, animal or vegetable, also referred as microorganism.

Microbial dietary adjuvant A substance added to the diet inorder to stimulate specific microbial processes and populations.

Microbial ecology The study of microorganisms in their natural environments, with a major emphasis on physical conditions, processes, and interactions, which occur on the scale of individual microbial cells.

Microbial loop The mineralization of organic matter synthesized by photosynthetic phytoplankton through the activity of microorganisms such as bacteria and protozoa and this process loops minerals and carbon dioxide back for reuse by the primary producers and makes the organic matter unavailable to higher consumers.

Microbial mat A firm structure of layered microorganisms with complementary physiological activities, which can develop on surfaces in aquatic environments.

Microbiology The study of microscopic life such as bacteria and viruses.

Microbivory The use of microorganisms as a food source by organisms, which can ingest or phagocytose them.

Microencapsulated Surrounded by a thin, protective layer of biodegradable substance referred as microsphere.

Micro-encapsulation Microencapsulation is a process by which solids, liquids, or gases are encased in microscopic capsules. Thin coatings of a wall material are formed around the substance to be encapsulated.

Microfilaments Protein filaments, about 4 to 7 nm in diameter, which are present in the cytoplasmic matrix of eucaryotic cells and play certain role in cell structure and motion.

Micromho A measure of conductance equal to one millionth of a mho.

Microinch A unit of length equal to one millionth of an inch (0.000001 inch).

Micron or micrometer A unit of length equal to one millionth of a meter (μm) or thousandth of a millimeter (25 μm are approximately 0.001 inch).

Micronucleus Refers to the smaller of the two nuclei in ciliate protozoa. It is diploid and involved only in genetic recombination and the regeneration of macronuclei.

Micronutrients Compounds essential for cellular growth, being present in concentrations less than about 1 mM in the growth medium, such as zinc, manganese, and copper that are required in very small quantities for growth and reproduction. They are also called trace elements.

Microorganism A microbe, a microscopic plant or animal, such as a bacterium, protozoan, yeast, virus, or alga (or) an organism that is too small to be seen clearly with the naked eye.

Microphyll A small leaf.

Microphyllidious Small, leaf-shaped.

Micropropagation Generation of new, disease free plants from tiny pieces of tissues.

Micropyle Refers to a small canal through the integument(s) at the apex of an ovule.

Microscopic diffusion control (encounter control) The observable consequence of the limitation that the rate of a bimolecular chemical reaction in a homogeneous medium cannot go beyond the rate of encounter of the reacting molecular entities.

Microsporangium Sporangium producing microspores, generally many in number, in the life cycle of a heterosporous plant.

Microtome An instrument used for cutting thin section of specimens.

Microtubules Small cylinders, about 25 nm in diameter, made of tubulin proteins, present in the cytoplasmic matrix and flagella of eucaryotic cells and are involved in cell structure and movement.

Microvilli Hair-like projections on the surface of the epithelial cells of the villi in the small intestine, which increase the surface area of the intestine to improve absorption of digested nutrients.

Midrib The central, and usually the most prominent, vein of a leaf or leaf-like organ.

Midbrain A network of neurons, which connects with the forebrain and relays sensory signals to other integrating centers.

Middle lamella A layer composed of pectin, which cements two adjoining plant cells together.

Migraine A condition, which is marked by recurrent, severe headaches on one side of the head and commonly associated with irritability, nausea, vomiting, constipation or diarrhea, and often sensitivity to light.

Miliary tuberculosis An acute form of tuberculosis in which small tubercles are formed in a number of organs of the body due to the dissemination of *M. tuberculosis* throughout the body by the bloodstream.

Milk of barium An aqueous suspension of barium hydroxide, $Ba(OH)_2$.

Milk of bismuth An aqueous suspension of basic bismuth nitrates, $Bi(OH)_2NO_3$ and/or $BiOH(NO_3)_2$

Milk of lime An aqueous suspension of calcium hydroxide, $Ca(OH)_2$.

Milk of magnesia An aqueous suspension of magnesium hydroxide, $Mg(OH)_2$.

Milk of sulfur Refers to precipitated sulfur.

Milk stage Refers to the early stage of grain development when the grain is filled with a milky liquid.

Milliequivalents The milliequivalent is the amount, in milligrams, of a solute equal to 1/1000 of its gram equivalent weight.

Milliosmoles Osmotic pressure is directly proportional to the total number of particles in solution.

The milliosmole is the unit of measure for osmotic concentration. For non-electrolytes, 1 millimole represents 1 milliosmole.

Mineralization The release of inorganic nutrients from organic matter during the microbial growth and metabolism.

Mineralocorticoids A group of steroid hormones that are produced by the adrenal cortex and are important in maintaining electrolyte balance.

Minerals Refer to trace elements required for normal metabolism, as components of cells and tissues, and in nerve conduction and muscle contraction.

Minienvironment The actual localized control space limited by a defined enclosure, which separates or isolates the inside from the outside environment, similar to the transfer of potential contamination from one side to the other is minimized or completely eliminated, depending on the design.

Minimal inhibitory concentration (MIC) The lowest concentration of a drug, which will prevent the growth of a particular microorganism.

Minimal lethal concentration (MLC) The lowest concentration of a drug, which will kill a particular microorganism.

Minituber Small tuber produced under greenhouse conditions on a small potato plant that is generated by micropropagation.

Minus, or negative, strand The virus nucleic acid strand, which is complementary in base sequence to the viral mRNA.

Missense mutation A single base substitution in DNA, which changes a codon for one amino acid into a codon for another.

Mitochondria Cytoplasmic organelles of most eukaryotic cells, known as the power house of energy, surrounded by a double membrane and produce adenosine 5'-triphosphate as useful energy for the cell by oxidative phosphorylation.

Mitochondrion The eucaryotic organelle, constructed of an outer membrane and an inner membrane, which contains the electron transport chain, which is the site of electron transport, oxidative phosphorylation, and pathways such as the Krebs cycle. It provides most of a nonphotosynthetic cell's energy under aerobic conditions.

Mitogen An agent or substance that stimulates mitosis (cell division) in lymphocytes.

Mitosis The process of nuclear division in cells, which produces daughter cells that are genetically identical to each other and to the parent cell.

Mitotic spindle Refers to a network of microtubules formed during prophase.

Mixed acid fermentation A type of fermentation in which ethanol and a complex mixture of organic acids are produced, which is carried out by members of the family Enterobacteriaceae.

Mixed airflow room Refers to a room which is supplied of air by conventional turbulent means, such as a diffuser or terminal HEPA filter, which also includes an unidirectional flow zone (such as a hood over a critical area). The total air changes of the room are enhanced by the operation of the hood.

Mixed-bed ion exchange Both anion and cation resins mixed in the same deionizer that results in higher efficiency, but lower capacity, than separate-bed deionizers.

Mixotrophic Refers to microorganisms that combine autotrophic and heterotrophic metabolic processes, use inorganic electron sources and organic carbon sources.

Mixture Composed of two or more substances, however, each keeps its original properties.

Mode The mode is the most frequently occurring value (or values) in a frequency distribution. The mode is useful for non-normal distributions especially bimodal distributions.

Modified atmosphere packaging (MAP) Addition of gases such as nitrogen and carbon dioxide to packaged foods in order to inhibit the growth of organisms that spoil the foods.

Moiety A part or portion of a molecule, generally complex, with a characteristic chemical or pharmacological property.

Moist air A binary mixture of dry air and water vapor in which each component behaves as if the other is not present and each occupies the complete volume of the mixture.

Moisturizer A combination of chemicals mixed together and applied to the skin, which can prevent the loss of skin water and thereby counteract dry, itchy skin.

Molality The number of moles of solute (the material dissolved) per kilogram of solvent (what the solute is dissolved in).

Molar An term expressing molarity, the number of moles of solute/ liters of solution.

Molarity The number of moles of solute (the material dissolved) per liter of solution, used to express the concentration of a solution.

Mold Any of a large group of fungi, which cause mold or moldiness and that exist as multicellular filamentous colonies. Molds characteristically do not produce macroscopic fruiting bodies.

Mole One gram molecular weight of a compound.

Mole fraction The number of moles of a particular substance that is expressed as a fraction of the total number of moles, or, it is the ratio of the number of moles of one component to the total moles of a mixture or solution.

Molecular chaperones Proteins, which aid in the proper folding of unfolded polypeptides or partly denatured proteins and also help transport proteins across membranes.

Molecular chronometers Nucleic acid and protein sequences, which gradually change over time in a random fashion and at a steady rate, and so it can be used to determine phylogenetic relationships.

Molecular entity Any chemically or isotopically distinct atom, molecule, ion, ion pair, radical, radical ion, complex, conformer, etc. that can be identified as a separately distinguishable entity.

Molecular formula Formula that shows the number of atoms of each element present in a molecule.

Molecular genetics Deals with the study of the nature and biochemistry of genetic material, also ncludes the technologies of genetic engineering.

Molecular geometry Shape of a molecule, based on the relative positions of the atoms.

Molecular graphics It is the visualization and manipulation of three-dimensional representations of molecules on a graphical display device.

Molecular metal Refers to a nonmetallic material whose properties resemble those of metals, generally following oxidative doping, e.g. polyacetylene following oxidative doping with iodine.

Molecular modeling A technique used for the investigation of molecular structures and properties using computational chemistry and graphical visualization techniques to provide a plausible three-dimensional representation under a given set of circumstances.

Molecular rearrangement The term is conventionally applied to any reaction, which involves a change of connectivity (sometimes including hydrogen), and violates the so-called "principle of minimum structural change". According to this oversimplified principle, chemical species do not isomerize in the course of a transformation, e.g. substitution, or the change of a functional group of a chemical species into a different functional group is not expected to involve the making or breaking of more than the minimum number of bonds required to affect that transformation.

Molecular weight The weight of a molecule, which may be calculated as the sum of the atomic weights of its constituent atoms, whereas, atomic weight is the weight of an element in relation to some element taken as the standard, usually oxygen (16) or carbon (12).

Molecularity The number of reactant molecular entities, which are involved in the microscopic chemical event constituting an elementary reaction.

Molecular biology Field of biology, which studies the molecular level of organization.

Molecule One molecule of any substance is the smallest physical unit of that particular substance.

Molish's reagent Reagent used for the detection of carbohydrates.

Moneocious Producing male and female gametes on the same individual

Monoamine-oxide Refers to a type of neurotransmitter.

Monoclonal antibody (Mab or MoAb) Antibodies derived from a single source or clone of cells, which recognize only one type of antigen, produced from hybridomas formed by the hybridization of two cells. A single antibody-producing cell and a cell that can be grown indefinitely in culture. Monoclonal antibodies have found markets in diagnostic kits and show potential for use in drugs and industrial purification processes.

Monocotyledons A class of angiosperms having an embryo with only one cotyledon, parts of the flower usually in threes, leaves with parallel veins, and scattered vascular bundles.

Monocytes White blood cells that clean up dead viruses, bacteria, and fungi and dispose of dead cells and debris at the end of the inflammatory response.

Monocyte-macrophage system The collection of fixed phagocytic cells, including macrophages, monocytes, and specialized endothelial cells, located in the liver, spleen, lymph nodes, and bone marrow. This system is an important component of the host's general nonspecific defense against pathogens.

Monokine A generic term for a cytokine that is produced by mononuclear phagocytes.

Monomer The basic subunit from which, by repetition of a single reaction, polymers are made, e.g. amino acids (monomers) condense to yield polypeptides or proteins (polymers).

Monosaccharides The building blocks of carbohydrates, hence known as simple sugar, classified by the number of carbon atoms in the molecule, pentoses have five and hexoses six. All monosaccharides, except dihydroxyacetone, possess chiral molecules, i.e. exhibiting stereoisomerism.

Monoterpene lactones Refer to iridoids.

Monoterpenoids With a base of $C_{10}H_{16}$, occur in essential oils and are made up of one or two isoprene rings or an open chain of isoprene units; colorless, water insoluble, volatile, with fragrant odour.

Morbidity rate Term that measures the number of individuals who become ill as a result of a particular disease within a susceptible population during a specific time period.

Morph Refers to a distinct phenotypic variant within a population.

Morphological convergence The evolution of basically dissimilar structures to serve a common function.

Morphology A branch of biology that deals with the form and structure of animals and plants, a study of the forms, relationships, metamorphoses, and phylogenetic development of organs apart from their functions.

Mortality rate The ratio of the number of deaths from a given disease to the total number of cases of the disease.

Mother liquor The residual liquid, which remains after the crystallization or isolation processes. A mother liquor may contain unrecovered products, (i.e. unreacted starting materials, intermediates, levels of the API and/or impurities), which may be used for further processing.

Motif A pattern of amino acids in a protein sequence with a specific function, e.g. metal binding.

Motor neurons Neurons, which receive signals from interneurons and transfer the signals to effector cells that produce a response.

Motor neuropathy Weakness initially felt in the arms, legs, hands, and feet resulting from damage to the nerves, which supply these areas of the body. Certain diseases and drug treatments can cause this problem.

Mottling Mottling is unequal color distribution, with light or dark areas standing out on an otherwise uniform surface.

Mouth The oral cavity, entrance to the digestive system where the food is broken into pieces by the teeth and saliva begins the process of digestion.

Mouthwashes Mouthwashes are solutions that are used to cleanse the mouth or treat diseases of the oral mucous membrane. They often contain alcohol or glycerin to aid in dissolving the volatile ingredients. Mouthwashes are more often used cosmetically than therapeutically.

MRI Abbreviation for magnetic resonance imaging, a diagnostic test, which is used to view images of the body without using X-rays.

MSDS (material safety data sheet) Document, originated by substance manufacturer, describing the chemical and physical properties of a substance as related to its safe handling and storage.

Mucilage A gelatinous substance, containing proteins and polysaccharides, which soothes inflammation.

Mucilaginous An herb or substance that is characterized by a gummy or gelatinous consistency which is soothing and healing to inflamed surfaces and mucous membranes

Mucociliary blanket The layer of cilia and mucus, which lines certain portions of the respiratory system, traps microorganisms up to 10 mm in diameter and then transports them by ciliary action away from the lungs.

Mucosal-associated lymphoid tissue The defensive immune lymphoid tissue, which is located in the intestinal mucosa.

Mucro A sharp, abrupt terminal point.

Mucus Refers to a thick, lubricating fluid that is produced by the mucous membranes, which line the respiratory, digestive, urinary and reproductive tracts. Also, serves as a barrier against infection and in the digestive tract, moistens food, making it easier to swallow.

Multicellular Refers to organisms composed of more than one cell.

Multicopper oxidases A group of enzymes, which oxidize organic substrates and reduce dioxygen to water.

Multi-drug-resistant strains of tuberculosis A multi-drug-resistant strain is defined as *Mycobacterium tuberculosis* resistant to isoniazid and rifampin, with or without resistance to other drugs.

Multienzyme A protein possessing more than one catalytic function that is contributed by distinct parts of a polypeptide chain (domains), or by distinct subunits, or both.

Multiheme Refers to a protein containing two or more heme groups.

Multiple sclerosis An autoimmune disease of the central nervous system, which includes the brain and spinal cord, MS affects the central nervous system by disrupting the conduction of electrical signals along neurons.

Multiplexing A sequencing approach, which uses several pooled samples simultaneously, greatly increasing sequencing speed.

Multi-use equipment Equipment that is used to process more than one product.

Mumps An acute generalized disease, which occurs primarily in school-age children and is caused by a paramyxovirus that is transmitted in saliva and respiratory droplets. The main manifestation is swelling of the parotid salivary glands.

Muricate With a rough surface texture owing to small, sharp projections.

Murine Relating to a member of the rodent family Muridae, including rats and mice, like murine monoclonal antibodies derived from mice.

Muscle tone A feature of muscle when it is under constant nerve stimulation.

Musculoskeletal system Refers to the bones, joints, muscles, tendons, and ligaments within the body.

Mutagen An agent, which induces cellular DNA to undergo mutation, e.g. X-rays.

Mutagenesis The induction of mutation in the genetic material of an organism, by physical or chemical means to improve the production of capabilities of organisms.

Mutant The altered cell that results from mutation of the original wild type or any subsequent alteration.

Mutarotation The change in optical rotation accompanying epimerisation.

Mutation An abrupt change of genotype that involves either the structure or number of complete chromosomes or, more commonly, a change in the structure of a single gene so that its function is altered or lost, certain chemicals called mutagens induce it.

Mutual prodrug A mutual prodrug is the connection in a unique mol-

ecule of two, usually synergistic, drugs attached to each other, one drug being the carrier for the other and vice versa.

Mutualism A type of symbiosis in that both the partners gain from the association and are unable to survive without it. The mutualist and the host are metabolically dependent on each other.

Mutualist An organism associated with another in a relationship that is beneficial to both.

Myalgia Aches and pains in muscles.

Mycelium A mass of branching hyphae found in fungi and some bacteria.

Mycobacterium A genus of the family Mycobacteriaceae that contains slender, aerobic, usually acid fast, gram-positive, rod-shaped organisms of various forms, club-shaped, swollen, but seldom branched or with filaments. It includes many species that were previously and are still called bacilli, such as the pathogens of tuberculosis and leprosy.

Mycobiont Refers to the fungal partner in a lichen.

Mycolic acids Complex 60 to 90 carbon fatty acids with a hydroxyl on the β-carbon and an aliphatic chain on the α-carbon, which is found in the cell walls of mycobacteria.

Mycologist A person specialized in mycology.

Mycology The science and study of fungi.

Mycoplasma Bacteria, which are members of the class Mollicutes and order Mycoplasmatales, lack cell walls and cannot synthesize peptidoglycan precursors, most require sterols for growth, the smallest, free-living organism with a size range from 1.25 μm to 0.5 μm.

Mycorrhiza Occurs when a fungus (basidiomycete or zygomycete) weaves around or into a plant's roots and forms a symbiotic relationship. Fungal hyphae absorb minerals from the soil and pass them to the plant roots while the fungus obtains carbohydrates from the plant.

Myelin A fatty insulating material that surrounds the axon.

Myeloma A malignant human plasma cell, which can synthesize excessive amounts of whole antibody or single immunoglobulin chains.

Myoglobin A monomeric dioxygen-binding hemeprotein of muscle tissue, which is structurally similar to a subunit of hemoglobin.

Myositis Inflammation of muscle tissue seen in diseases such as dermatomyositis and polymyositis.

Myotic Cause the contraction of the pupil and diminution of ocular tension.

Myricetin Refers to a common flavonol.

Myristic acid A saturated 14-carbon fatty acid, $CH_3 (CH_2)_{12} COOH$, that occurs in many fats.

Myrosinase The enzyme that breaks down glucosinolates, yielding distinctive isothiocyanates.

Myxobacteria A group of gram-negative, aerobic soil bacteria that is characterized by gliding motility, a complex life cycle with the production of fruiting bodies, and the formation of myxospores.

Myxospores Special dormant spores that are formed by the myxobacteria.

N

NAA Naphthalene acetic acid, a synthetic auxin which is very useful in stimulating rooting in cuttings and promoting flowering.

NAD⁺ Oxidized form of nicotinamide adenine dinucleotide, despite the plus sign in the symbol, the coenzyme is anionic under normal physiological conditions.

NADH Reduced form of nicotinamide adenine dinucleotide.

NADP⁺ Oxidized form of nicotinamide adenine dinucleotide phosphate, despite the plus sign in the symbol, the coenzyme is anionic under normal physiological conditions.

NADPH Reduced form of nicotinamide adenine dinucleotide phosphate.

Naked Lacking hairs or scales.

Naphthoquinones Pigments, quinones in which a second aromatic ring is fused to the benzoquinone ring, occurring as free glycosides.

Napkin (diaper) candidiasis Usually found in infants whose diapers are not changed frequently and are therefore not kept dry, caused by Candida species of fungi.

Narcissistic reaction A chemical reaction, which can be described as the conversion of a reactant into its mirror image, without rotation or translation of the product, so that the product enantiomer actually coincides with the mirror image of the reactant molecule.

Narcotic An herb or substance that will relieve pain and induce sleep when used in medicinal doses.

Narrow-spectrum drugs Chemotherapeutic agents, which are effective only against a limited variety of microorganisms.

Nasal sprays They are used for the nasal delivery of a drug or drugs, generally to alleviate cold or allergy symptoms such as nasal congestion.

National Formulary (NF) A compendium of purity and testing criteria for chemicals, usually used in combination with the USP.

Native species Refers to a species that occurs naturally in a particular geographic area.

Natural attenuation Decrease in the level of an enviromental contaminant, which results from natural chemical, physical, and biological processes.

Natural classification A classification system, which arranges organisms into groups whose members share many characteristics and reflect as much as possible the biological nature of organisms.

Natural flavor The term natural flavor or natural flavoring means the essential oil, oleoresin, essence or extractive, protein hydrolysate, distillate, or any product of roasting, heating or enzymolysis, which contains the flavoring constituents derived from a spice, fruit or fruit juice, vegetable or vegetable juice, edible yeast, herb, bark, bud, root, leaf or similar plant material, meat, seafood, poultry, eggs, dairy products, or fermentation products thereof, whose significant function in food is flavoring rather than nutritional.

Natural killer (NK) cell A non-T, non-B lymphocyte present in nonimmunized individuals, which exhibits MHC-independent cytolytic activity against tumor cells.

Naturalized species An alien species, which has been introduced to an area and has adapted to the growing conditions of that area, so that it is able to survive and reproduce without human assistance or cultivation.

Naturally acquired active immunity The type of active immunity that develops when an individual's immunologic system comes into contact with an appropriate antigenic stimulus during the course of normal activities, usually arises as the result of recovering from an infection and lasts a long time.

Naturally acquired passive immunity The type of temporary immunity, which involves the transfer of antibodies from one individual to another.

Naturopathy A form of health care system that uses diet, herbs, and other natural methods and substances to cure illness without the use of drugs.

Nauseant An herb or substance that produces vomiting and nausea.

Necrosis The pathological death of one or more cells, or of a portion of tissue or organ, resulting from irreversible damage to the nucleus. In leaves, death of tissue accompanied by dark brown discoloration, usually occurring in a well-defined part of a plant, such as the portion of a leaf between leaf veins or the xylem or phloem in a stem or tuber.

Necrotizing fasciitis Necrotizing fasciitis is an infection of the subcutaneous soft tissues, particularly of fibrous tissue, and is most common on the extremities. The infection begins with skin reddening, swelling, pain, and cellulitis, and proceeds to skin breakdown and gangrene after 3 to 5 days.

Necrotroph Refers to the parasite that kills the host cells, so being essentially saprophytic in its nutrition.

Nectar Refers to the sweetish liquid in many flowers used by bees for the making of honey.

Nectary A part of a flower that secretes nectar.

Negative staining A staining procedure in that a dye is used to make the background dark while the specimen is unstained.

Negri bodies Masses of viruses or unassembled viral subunits, which are found within the brain neurons of rabies-infected animals.

Neoflavonoids Flavonoids in which ring B is attached to C-4 or as 4-phenylcoumarins.

Neoplasm Any new growth of cells or tissues and the term is usually used to constantly progressive, comparatively unlimited, or uncontrolled new growth that manifests varying degrees of autonomy.

Nephelometer Any apparatus that is used to measure the size and concentration of particles in a liquid by analysis of light transmitted through or reflected by the liquid.

Nephelometry The semiquantitative estimation of the concentration of particles in a suspension, by comparing it with the standard suspensions in a nephelometer.

Nephron A tubular structure, which is the functional unit of the kidney, consists of a glomerulus and renal tubule.

Nephrotoxin A cytotoxin, which is specific for cells of the kidney.

Nerve A bundle of neurons responsible for the conduction of electrical impulses in the body.

Nerve conduction Refers to the passage of electrical impulses through nerves in the body.

Nervine An herb or substance that relaxes, soothes, calms, and quiets the nerves, or which acts on the entire nervous system in a beneficial manner to allay nervous excitement.

Nervous system A system containing all the nerve systems in the body that includes the brain, spinal cord, and the series of nerves throughout the body.

Neurologist A physician specialized in the diagnosis and treatment of disorders of the nervous system.

Neurons The building blocks or basic nerve cells of the nervous system.

Neuropathy Numbness, tingling, and/or weakness initially felt in the arms, legs, hands, and feet resulting from damage to the nerves, which supply sensation to these areas of the body. Certain diseases and drug treatments cause this problem.

Neurotoxin A toxin, which is poisonous to or destroys nerve tissue, especially the toxins secreted by *C. tetani*, *Corynebacterium diphtheriae* and *Shigella dysenteriae*.

Neurotransmitters Refer to chemicals released from the tip of an axon into the synaptic cleft when a nerve impulse arrives. They may stimulate or inhibit the next neuron.

Neustonic The microorganisms, which live at the atmospheric interface of a water body.

Neutral An object, which does not have a positive or negative charge.

Neutral flower Sterile flower composed of a perianth without any sexual organs.

Neutron A particle found in the nucleus of an atom, almost identical in mass to a proton, but carries no electric charge.

Neutrophil A mature white blood cell in the granulocyte lineage, which is formed in bone marrow, has a nucleus with three to five lobes and is very phagocytic.

Neutrophile Refers to microorganisms that grow best at a neutral pH range between pH 5.5 and 8.0.

New chemical entity A new chemical entity (NCE) is a compound that is not previously described in the literature.

New drug application (NDA) The new drug application contains most of the information included in the IND (investigational new drug), submitted to FDA and only after FDA approval of the NDA, distribution and marketing of a new drug begin.

New indication A therapeutic use for a pharmaceutical product which has been discovered and developed after the product's initial marketing authorisation.

NHSA (normal human serum albumin) A blood plasma fraction usually prepared by Cohn cold ethanol precipitation, dispensed as a 5 to 25% protein solution.

Niche The function of an organism in a complex system that includes place of the organism, the resources used in a given location and the time of use.

Nicotinamide adenine dinucleotide An electron-carrying coenzyme, particularly important in catabolic processes and usually donates its electrons to the electron transport chain under aerobic conditions.

Nicotinamide adenine dinucleotide phosphate An electron-carrying coenzyme, which most often participates as an electron carrier in biosynthetic metabolism.

Nicotine A pyridine alkaloid.

Nif A set of about 20 genes that are required for the assembly of the nitrogenase enzyme complex.

Ninhydrin reagent Reagent used for the detection of amino acid.

Nitrate reductase A metalloenzyme, containing molybdenum, which reduces nitrate to nitrite.

Nitrification Refers to the oxidation of ammonia to nitrate.

Nitrifying bacteria Chemolithotrophic, gram-negative bacteria, members of the family Nitrobacteriaceae and convert ammonia to nitrate and nitrite to nitrate.

Nitrite reductase A metalloenzyme, which reduces nitrite, dissimilatory nitrite reductases contain copper and reduce nitrite to nitrogen monoxide, assimilatory nitrite reductases contain siroheme and iron-sulfur clusters and reduce nitrite to ammonia.

Nitrogen fixation The assimilation of dinitrogen by microbial reduction to ammonia and conversion into organonitrogen compounds such as amino acids. Only a limited number of microorganisms are able to fix nitrogen.

Nitrogen oxygen demand (NOD) The demand for oxygen in sewage treatment that is caused by nitrifying microorganisms.

Nitrogen saturation point Refers to the point at which mineral nitrogen, when added to an ecosystem, can no longer be incorporated into organic matter through biological processes.

Nitrogenase The enzyme, which catalyzes biological nitrogen fixation.

Nitrogenous anthocyanins Refers to betalains.

Nitrogenous base A nitrogen containing molecule, which has the chemical properties of a base.

Nm An abbreviation for nanometers. A nanometer is equal to 10^{-9} meters.

Nocardioforms Bacteria that resemble members of the genus Nocardia, they develop a substrate mycelium, which readily breaks up into rods and coccoid elements.

Nocturia The need to urinate during the night.

Nocturnal Flowers, opening only at night.

Node Refers to a knob or joint of a stem from which leaves, roots, shoots, or flowers may arise. It will contain one or more buds.

Nomenclature The making and giving distinguishing names to all groups of plants (or) the branch of taxonomy concerned with the assignment of names to taxonomic groups in agreement with published rules.

Nominal pore size Based on retention efficiency, a filter should retain 99.9% of particles larger than its nominal rated pore size.

Nominal outside diameter A numerical identification of outside diameter to which tolerances apply.

Nominal wall thickness A numerical identification of wall thickness to which tolerances apply.

Non-articulated Laticifer, lacking cross walls.

Nonbonded interactions Intramolecular attractions or repulsions between atoms, which are not directly linked to each other, affecting the thermodynamic stability of the chemical species concerned.

Noncarbonate hardness Hardness in water caused by chlorides, sulfates, and nitrates of calcium and magnesium.

Nonclassical carbocation Refers to a carbocation, the ground state of which has delocalized (bridged) bonding pi- or sigma-electrons.

Noncompliance Nonadherent, not staying on a specific regimen.

Noncyclic photophosphorylation The process in which light energy is used to make ATP when electrons are moved from water to NADP1 during photosynthesis, both photosystem I and photosystem II are involved.

Non-electrolytes Non-electrolytes are substances that do not form ions when dissolved in water. Examples are estradiol, glycerin, urea, and sucrose.

Non-GMP technology Facility design requirement that results from decisions to address issues outside the realm of GMPs or manufacturer preferences. These affect GMP related design features.

Nongonococcal urethritis (NGU) Any inflammation of the urethra not caused by *Neisseria gonorrhoeae*.

Non-hydrolysable tannins Proanthocyanidins.

Non-naturalized species An alien species, which is capable of growing with assistance or cultivation, but does not successfully reproduce and disperse in the wild. These plants usually do not persist without being replanted on a regular basis.

Nonpolar Nonpolar molecules that have perfect symmetry have dipole moments of zero.

Non-protein amino acids Refers to amino acids not associated with proteins, many important in the storage and transport of soluble nitrogen, often present in large quantities in seeds, sometimes poisonous.

Nonsense codon A codon, which does not code for an amino acid but is a signal to terminate protein synthesis.

Nonsense mutation A mutation, which converts a sense codon to a nonsense or stop codon.

Nonspecific resistance Refers to those general defense mechanisms that are inherited as part of the innate structure and function of each animal. It is also known as nonspecific, innate or natural immunity.

Nonunidirectional airflow Air distribution where the first air entering the controlled space mixes with the internal air by means of induction. The airflow, which does not meet the definition of unidirectional airflow is referred as turbulent or non-laminar airflow.

Nonvascular plants Plants lacking lignified vascular tissue (xylem), vascularized leaves, and having a free-living, photosynthetic gametophyte stage that dominates the life cycle, e.g. mosses and liverworts.

Norepinephrine A hormone produced in the adrenal medulla that is secreted under stress.

Normal microbiota Microorganisms normally associated with a particular tissue or structure.

Normal saline 0.9 % w/v of sodium chloride in water.

Normality A convenient way of dealing with acids, bases, and electrolytes involves the use of equivalents. One equivalent of an acid is the quantity of that acid that supplies or donates one mole of H, ions. One equivalent of a base is the quantity that furnishes one mole of OH^- ions. One equivalent of acid reacts with one equivalent of base. The normality (N) of a solution is the number of gram-equivalent weights (equivalents) of solute per liter of solution.

Northern blot A recombinant DNA technique, which is used for the detection of specific RNA transcripts.

Nosode A homeopathic remedy made from diseased tissue or bodily secretions rather than from a plant or animal that is taken like a homeopathic immunization to build up an immune response against a specific disease. They are often named for the disease present in the material they were made from, e.g. the flu nosode and the infectious mononucleosis nosode.

Not exposed or closed Drug substance is protected from exposure to the environment during processing.

Noxious weed A weed that is specified by law as being especially undesirable, troublesome and difficult to control.

NPDWR water Refers to potable water meeting EPA National Primary Drinking Water Regulations.

Nucellar beak A structure in the ovule where nucellar tissue protrudes through the micropyle.

Nucellus In plants, it refers to the watery tissue composing the chief part of the young ovule in the flower and inside the seed during early development or the central tissue of an ovule of a seed plant. It furnishes nutrients to the young embryo and is digested by the developing endosperm and embryo.

Nuclear area A region containing the cell's genetic information in prokaryotic cells.

Nuclear magnetic resonance (NMR) spectroscopy NMR spectroscopy makes it possible to distinguish nuclei, typically protons, in different chemical environments.

Nuclear Refers to endosperm formation, where nuclear divisions are at least initially not accompanied by cell wall formation, a syncytium being formed.

Nuclearity The number of central atoms joined in a single coordination entity by bridging ligands or metal-metal bonds is indicated by dinuclear, trinuclear, tetranuclear, polynuclear, etc.

Nuclease Refers to an enzyme, which breaks down nucleic acids. Exonucleases cleave the nucleotides only at the ends of polynucleotide chains (e.g. phosphodiesterase). Endonucleases attack certain linkages wherever they occur in the polynucleotide chain.

Nucleation The process by which nuclei are formed, usually in solution, the term nucleus as used here is defined as the smallest solid phase aggregate of atoms, molecules or ions that is formed during a precipitation and which is capable of spontaneous growth.

Nucleic acid A large molecule composed of nucleotide subunits (or) the non-protein constituents of nucleo-protiens, have a high molecular weight and consists of alternate units of phosphate and a pentose sugar, which has a purine and pyrimidine base attached to it.

Nucleic acid hybridization Matching of either DNA or RNA, depending on the organism, from an unknown organism with DNA or RNA from a known organism. This method is used in disease research for identifying species and strains of organisms.

Nucleocapsid Refers to the nucleic acid and its surrounding protein coat or capsid, the basic unit of virion structure.

Nucleoid The compact body, which contains the genome in a bacterium.

Nucleolus A discrete region of the nucleus that is created by the transcription of rRNA genes. The nucleolus disappears during mitosis, or cell division.

Nucleophile, nucleophilic A nucleophile (or nucleophilic reagent) is a reagent, which forms a bond to its reaction partner (the electrophile) by donating both bonding electrons.

Nucleoside Refers to a combination of ribose or deoxyribose with a purine or pyrimidine base.

Nucleosome A complex of histones and DNA, which is found in eucaryotic chromatin, the DNA is wrapped around the surface of the beadlike histone complex.

Nucleotide The structural unit of nucleic acids, subunit of DNA or RNA consisting of purine bases (adenine, guanine), pyrimidine bases (thymine, or cytosine in DNA; uracil, or cytosine in RNA), a phosphate molecule, and a sugar molecule (deoxyribose in DNA and ribose in RNA). Thousands of nucleotides are linked to form a DNA or RNA molecule.

Nucleotide sequences The genetic code that is encrypted in the sequence of bases along a nucleic acid.

Nucleus The cellular organelle present in eukaryote cells and separated from the cytoplasm by a nuclear membrane, contains the genetic material and is essential for the continued life of the cell.

Numbness A loss of the sensation of feeling.

Numerical aperture The property of a microscope lens, which determines how much light can enter and how great a resolution the lens can provide.

Numerical taxonomy The grouping by numerical methods of taxonomic units into taxa based upon their character states.

Numerous Many.

Nut A hard, dry, indehiscent fruit that is formed from two or more carpels but containing only one seed.

Nutlet A small nut.

Nutraceuticals Any substance that may be considered as food or part of food which in addition to its normal nutritive value, provides health benefits including prevention of disease.

Nutrient An herb or substance that affects the nutritive processes and metabolic changes in the body, supplies material for tissue building, contains necessary food values such as vitamins and minerals, or which acts to release these elements from other food which has already been eaten but not assimilated.

Nutritive cell Refers to a specific cell of carpogonial branch with which carpogonium fuses after fertilization in some red algae of the order Cryptonemiales.

Nutritive Same as nutrient.

Nystagmus Involuntary, rapid movements of the eyes.

O

O antigen A polysaccharide antigen that extends from the outer membrane of some gram-negative bacterial cell walls. It is part of the lipopolysaccharide.

Oblanceolate Shaped like a lance point reversed, i.e. having the tapering point next to the leafstalk.

Obligate aerobes Organisms, which grow only in the presence of oxygen.

Obligate anaerobes Microorganisms, which cannot tolerate the presence of oxygen and die when exposed to it.

Oblique Slanting, unequal sided.

Oblong Elliptical and from two to four times as long as broad.

Obovate Inversely ovate, with the shape of the longitudinal section of an egg, with the broad end at the top, as some leaves.

Obovoid Inversely ovoid, roughly egg-shaped, with narrow end downwards, referes to some fruits.

Obsolescent Non-functional but not reduced to a rudiment.

Obsolete Reduced to a rudiment, or completely lacking.

Obturator A outgrowth of the funicle (commonest), placenta, or integument, etc. that forms a bridge between the micropyle and other tissues and is believed to faciltate fertilisation.

Obtuse With blunt or rounded end.

Occipital lobe The lobe of the cerebral cortex that is located at the rear of the head, which is responsible for receiving and processing visual information.

Occupational therapy Therapy that assists patients in their daily activities, including dressing, bathing, grooming, meal preparation, writing, and housework.

Ocean The great body of salt water, which covers mores than two-thirds of the surface of the earth.

Ocrea A tube-like covering around some stems.

Octet In Lewis structures, the objective is to make almost all atoms have an octet. This means that they will have access to 8 electrons regularly, even if they do have to share some of them.

Odontopathogens Dental pathogens.

O-glycosyl When the sugar is attached to the aglycone by a – O- bond.

Ohm Unit of electrical resistance in a circuit, such that a potential difference of one volt across a load of one ohm produces a current of one ampere.

Oils Fatty acid and glycerol or triglycerides that are liquid at room temperature.

Ointment It is a viscous semisolid preparation used topically on a variety of body surfaces.

Okazaki fragments Short stretches of polynucleotides that are produced during discontinuous DNA replication.

Oleaginous bases Oleaginous bases are anhydrous and insoluble in water. They cannot absorb or contain water and are not washable in water.

Oleo-gum-resin Oleoresin and gum in homogenous mixture.

Oleoresin A homogenous mixture of resin(s) and volatile oil(s).

Oleoside A type of secoiridoid monoterpene.

Oleum Refers to the fixed oil preparation pressed or squeezed from the plant material.

Oligomeric Oligo means short, refers to a type of polymer with only a few subunits, as opposed to a 'monomer' with one unit, or a 'polymer' with many subunits.

Oligonucleotide Macromolecules composed of short sequences of nucleotides, which are usually synthetically prepared and used.

Oligosaccharide Refers to any carbohydrate which is having 2-10 polymerized monosaccharide units. It is mostly having two (disaccharides), three (trisaccharides) or four (tetrasaccharides) sugar units. These may act as intermediates in polysaccharide metabolism or may serve as storage products.

Oligotrophic environment An environment that contains low levels of nutrients, particularly nutrients that support microbial growth.

Oncogene A gene whose activity is linked with the conversion of normal cells to cancer cells.

Onium ion A cation (with its counterion) that is derived by addition of a hydron to a mononuclear parent hydride of the nitrogen, chalcogen and halogen family, e.g. H_4N^+ ammonium ion.

Ontogeny The development of a single organism, i.e. the series of morphologies through which it passes during its lifetime.

Onychomycosis A fungal infection of the nail plate producing nails that are opaque, white, thickened, friable, and brittle, also called ringworm of the nails and tinea unguium, caused by Trichophyton and other fungi such as *C. albicans*.

Oocyst Cyst that is formed around a zygote of malaria and related protozoa.

Oogenesis The production of ova.

Oogonia Mitotically dividing female structures that produce primary oocytes and gametes.

Open meristem Refers to a root apical meristem in which all the tissue regions of the root can be traced to a single group of initials/cells.

Operating parameter Any information entered into an automated system, which is used for automated equipment operation. Or, a parameter indicative of the operating condition of a system.

Operating range The validated acceptance criteria within which a control parameter must remain, wherein acceptable product is being manufactured.

Operculum A distincly delimited and thickened ectexinous or sexinous structure, which covers part of an ectoaperture of a pollen grain.

Operon A functional unit consisting of a promoter, an operator and a number of structural genes, mainly found in prokaryotes.

Ophthalmia neonatorum A gonorrheal eye infection in a newborn that may lead to blindness, also called conjunctivitis of the newborn.

Ophthalmics Pertaining to products for the eyes. GMP requirements for the preparation of ophthalmics are essentially identical to those for parenterals.

Opposite Of leaves or bracts occurring two at a node on opposite sides of the stem.

Optic neuritis A change in the optic nerves because of demyelination of the nerve fibers.

Optical activity A sample of material able to rotate the plane of polarisation of a beam of transmitted plane-polarised light is said to possess optical activity.

Optical purity The ratio of the observed optical rotation of a sample consisting of a mixture of enantiomers to the optical rotation of one pure enantiomer.

Optically detected magnetic resonance (ODMR) A double resonance technique in which transitions between spin sublevels are detected by optical means. Generally, these are sublevels of a triplet, and the transitions are induced by microwaves.

Optically labile Term that describes a system in which stereoisomerisation results in a change of optical rotation with time.

Oral Relating to the mouth.

Oral product A pharmaceutical product meant to be introduced through the mouth in the form of a tablet, capsule, or suspension.

Oral solid dosage drug Formulated in a solid or powder form for patient to ingest orally.

Orbicular Round or shield-shaped with petiole attached to center.

Orbicular Circular or nearly so.

Orbicules Minute granules of sporopollenin secreted by the tapetum, occasionally found on pollen grains.

Orbital steering A concept expressing that the stereochemistry of approach of two reacting species is governed by the most favourable overlap of their appropriate orbitals.

Orbital symmetry The behaviour of an atomic or localized molecular orbital under molecular symmetry operations characterizes its orbital symmetry.

Orbitals An energy state in the atomic model that describes where an electron will likely be.

Orchitis Inflammation of the testes.

Order In the taxonomic hierarchy, a monophyletic grouping of families, or sometimes a single family with no apparent close relatives, the name with a termination ales, the major taxonomic rank between family and class.

Organ culture Refers to culture of excised organs, e.g. roots, leaves, embryos, meristerms, etc. in a suitable aseptic medium.

Organelle Used for describing any of the membrane-bound structures that are present in the cytoplasm of a cell. It is for carrying out a specific metabolic process essential to the life of cell, e.g. mitochondrion, chloroplast, etc.

Organic In chemistry, any carbon-containing compound is said to be organic.

Organism An individual, composed of organ systems, if multicellular.

Organogenesis Refers to developmental changes that take

place during formation of a particular organ.

Organosulfides The mostly smelly compounds in the allium (onion-garlic) and cruciferous (broccoli-kale) families.

Organosulfur Refers to an organic compound containing sulfur.

Organotrophs Organisms, which use reduced organic compounds as their electron source.

Originator medicinal product The first version of a medicinal product, developed and patented by an originator pharmaceutical company that receives exclusive rights to marketing the product in the European Union for 15 years.

Orobanchoside A phenylpropanoid, an ester of caffeic acid, two molecules and two sugar molecules also being involved.

Orphan drug The FDA grants orphan drug status to one company for a drug which is believed to substantially increase the life expectancy of the treated patient for a particular disease. This excludes other companies from receiving an FDA license to produce a similar drug for a finite period (usually 7 years), thereby allowing the company producing the drug to recuperate their R&D expenses.

Orthomolecular medicine A form of nutrient therapy, which uses combinations of vitamins, minerals, and amino acids normally found in the body to maintain good health and to treat specific conditions, such as asthma, heart disease, depression, and schizophrenia. Orthomolecular refres to an approach based on a correct (ortho) balance of substances present in the body.

Orthotropic Refers to growth, negatively geotropic, i.e. the stem growing more or less erect.

Orthotropous Atropous (of an ovule).

Osmophilic microorganisms Microorganisms, which grow best in or on media of high solute concentration.

Osmoregulation The regulation of the movement of water by osmosis into and out of cells. Also, the maintenance of water balance within the body.

Osmosis The diffusion of a solvent through a semipermeable membrane from a solution of higher concentration to one of lower concentration until there are equal concentrations of fluid on both sides of the membrane.

Osmotic potential Solute potential, symbol ψ_p said of the decrease in water potential of a solution in water which occurs due to dissolved ionic or non-ionic solute particle in it or the decrease in chemical potential of solvent in a solution which occurs due to presence of ionic or non-ionic solute particles.

Osmotic pressure The pressure which is developed due to the passage of water by osmosis. The maximum osmotic pressure of a given solution is developed when it is separated from pure water by a semi-permeable membrane.

Osmotolerant organisms That grow over a fairly wide range of water activity or solute concentration.

Ossification Refers to the process by which embryonic cartilage is replaced with bone.

Osteoblasts Refer to bone-forming cells.

Osteoporosis A disorder in that the minerals leach out of the bones, rendering them progressively more porous and fragile.

Ostiole An opening or pore, e.g. of a microsporangium or anther as it dehisces (little used in flowering plants), or at the apex of a fig.

Outbreak The sudden, unexpected occurrence of a disease in a given population.

Outer bark In older trees, the dead part of the bark.

Outer membrane Refers to a special membrane located outside the peptidoglycan layer in the cell walls of gram-negative bacteria.

Ovary In flowering plants, the part of the flower that encloses the ovules, when the ovary matures, it becomes the fruit. In animals, the female gonads, which produce eggs and female sex hormones.

Ovate With the shape of a longitudinal section of an egg; egg-shaped and attached by the broader end.

Oviparous Egg-laying, producing eggs that hatch after leaving the body of the female, germinating while still attached to the parent plant.

Oviposit To lay or deposit eggs.

Ovoid Egg-shaped.

Ovotransferrin An iron-binding protein from eggs, which is structurally similar to the transferrins.

Ovule In seed plants, the structure which gives rise to the seed.

Ovule culture Refers to the culture of excised ovules on suitable media in vitro for purpose of study or plant propagation.

Ovuliferous That bears ovules, e.g. applied to scales in a mega-sporangiate cone in gymnosperms.

Ovum Egg.

Oxalic acid A common organic acid in plants, oxalate itself is usually found in plants as calcium oxalate.

Oxidase An enzyme which catalyzes the oxidation of substrates by O_2.

Oxidation/reduction Oxidation means adding an atom of oxygen or removing an atom of hydrogen from a molecule, where as reduction means removing an oxygen atom or adding a hydrogen atom to a molecule.

Oxidation number The oxidation number of an element in any chemical entity is the number of charges which would remain on a given atom if the pairs of electrons in each bond to that atom were assigned to the more electronegative member of the bond pair. The oxidation (stock) number of an element is indicated by a roman numeral placed in parentheses immediately following the name (modified if necessary by an appropriate ending) of the element to which it refers (or) a number assigned to each atom to help keep track of the electrons during a redox-reaction.

Oxidation reaction A reaction where a substance loses electrons.

Oxidation-reduction (redox) reactions Reactions involving electron transfers, reductant donates electrons to an oxidant.

Oxidative addition The insertion of a metal of a coordination entity into a covalent bond that involves formally an overall two-electron loss on one metal or a one-electron loss on each of two metals.

Oxidative phosphorylation Refers to the synthesis of ATP from ADP using energy made available during electron transport.

Oxidizing agent or oxidant The electron acceptor in an oxidation-reduction reaction.

Oxidoreductase An enzyme that catalyzes an oxidation-reduction reaction.

Oxyacid When one or more hydroxide (OH) groups are bonded to a central atom.

Oxygen-evolving complex (OEC) The enzyme that catalyzes the formation of O_2 in photosynthesis.

Oxygenic photosynthesis Photosynthesis, which oxidizes water to form oxygen; the form of photosynthesis characteristic of eucaryotic algae and cyanobacteria.

Ozone It is formed by an electric discharge or by the slow combustion of phosphorus, ozone is a modified and condensed form of oxygen, in which three atoms of oxygen are combined to form the molecule, O_3. Since it is a powerful oxidizing agent, it is used in deionized water systems to kill bacteria and to reduce by oxidation the amount of total organic carbon (TOC) in the water. Air containing a perceptible amount of ozone has an odor suggesting chlorine or sulfurous acid gas.

P

Pacemaker enzyme The enzyme in a metabolic pathway, which catalyzes the slowest or rate-limiting reaction, if its rate changes, the pathway's activity changes.

Pachycaul Refers to trees, with particularly stout trunk and branches.

Packaging All operations, including filling and labeling that a bulk product has to undergo in order to become a finished product.

Packaging material Any material that is intended to protect an intermediate or API (active pharmaceutical ingredient) during storage and transport.

Palea The upper, and usually shorter and thinner, of two membranous bracts that encloses the flower in grasses.

Paleoherb Any member of a group of basal flowering herbs that may be the closest relatives of the monocots.

Palisade layer A layer of elongated cells that is set at right angles to the surface of a leaf or thallus and is underlying the upper epidermis or layers of cells. Its cells have numerous chloroplasts and is concerned with photosynthesis.

Palisade tissue One or more layers of palisade cells beneath the epidermis of a leaf.

Palisade Especially of leaf mesophyll, but of tissues in general, where the cells are elongated, closely packed, and upright.

Palmate Leaves divided into lobes arising from a common center (palm).

Palmatifid Refers to leaf, deeply (but not completely) divided into several lobes which arise (almost) at the same level.

Palmatisect A condition intermediate between palmate and palmatifid, with the green tissue of the lamina completely divided into several segments, but the segments not fully separated at the base.

Palmitic acid A 16-carbon saturated fatty acid found in most fats and oils, particularly associated with stearic acid.

Palynology The scientific study of pollen.

Pancreas A gland in the abdominal cavity, which secretes digestive enzymes into the small intestine and also secretes the hormones insulin and glucagon into the blood, where they regulate blood glucose levels. A digestive organ that produces trypsin, chymotrypsin and other enzymes as a pancreatic juice, but which also has endocrine functions in the production of the hormones somatostatin, insulin, and glucagon.

Pancreatic islets Clusters of endocrine cells in the pancreas, which secrete insulin and glucagons, also known as islets of Langerhans.

Pandemic disease An epidemic over an especially wide geographic area.

Pandurate Of leaves, shaped somewhat like a violin, as some leaves.

Paneth cell The granular cell located at the base of glands in the small intestine, produces the enzyme lysozyme.

Panicle A branched racemose inflorescence often applied more widely to any branched inflorescence.

Paniculate Panicled, arranged or growing in panicles.

Pannus Refers to a superficial vascularization of the cornea with infiltration of granulation tissue.

Panzootic The wide dissemination of a disease in an animal population.

Papilla A glandular hair with one secreting cell above the epidermis level.

Papillose Descriptive of a surface beset with short, blunt, rounded, or cylindric projections.

Pappus The modified calyx of flowers in the sunflower family, generally takes the form of bristles, scales, or awns.

Papverine An isoquinoline alkaloid.

Papyraceous Such as parchment in texture.

PAR (proven acceptable range) A range for a critical parameter that has been determined to be achievable and appropriate for the process or processes with which it is associated, established by knowledge gained through relevant documentation and actual testing. A process should perform consistently and as intended when all critical parameters are held within the established PARs.

Paracarpous Refers to a syncarpous gynoecium where the carpellary units are congenitally united only by their margins, the placentation thus being parietal.

Paracellular transport Drug transport across tight (narrow) junctions between cells or trans-enclothelial channels of cells is known as paracellular transport.

Paraclade Lateral branches of a synflorescence that has the same structure as the whole inflorescence.

Paracytic Refers to stomata, with two cells surrounding and parallel to the guard cells.

Parallel Of leaf venation, as used in the descriptions a general term for leaves in which there are several veins approximately equal in prominence that run more or less parallel the length of the blade, whether initially recurved or not or converging at the apex of the blade or not.

Parallelocytic Refers to stomata, with an alternating complex of three or more C-shaped subsidiary cells of graded sizes parallel to guard cells.

Paralysis The inability to move a part of the body.

Paralytic shellfish poisoning Dinoflagellates (Gonyaulax spp.) produce a powerful neurotoxin called saxitoxin. Shellfish accumulates saxitoxin and is poisonous when consumed by animals and humans. Saxitoxin paralyzes the striated respiratory muscles by inhibiting sodium transport.

Paramagnetic Substances having a positive magnetic susceptibility are paramagnetic. They are attracted by a magnetic field.

Parapatric Refers to distributions of two taxa or populations, having non-overlapping but contiguous ranges.

Paraphyletic A taxon made up of members which, given a particular phylogenetic tree and classification based on it, include only but not all the descendents a common ancestor, likely to be a grade.

Parasite An organism, which derives its food from the body of another organism, the host, without killing the host directly, also an insect that spends its immature stages in the body of a host that dies just before the parasite emerges.

Parasiticide Destroys parasites.

Parasitism A type of symbiosis in which one organism adversely affects the other (the host), but cannot live without it.

Parasorbic acid Refers to a lactone.

Parastichy A spiral linking primordia by some constant in their order of development.

Parasympathetic system The subdivision of the autonomic nervous system, which reverses the effects of the sympathetic nervous system, controls heartbeat, respiration and other vital functions.

Paratracheal Of axial parenchyma, associated with the vessels.

Parenchyma A generalized cell or tissue in a plant. These cells may manufacture or store food, and can often divide or differentiate into other kinds of cells. Air spaces are often present and the tissue is often for storage.

Parenchyma sheath A parenchymatous, single layered bundle sheath surrounding a vascular bundle, homologous to the endodermis.

Parent compound Refers to a compound from which other compounds are derived.

Parent isotope An element, which undergoes nuclear decay.

Parenteral drug (LVP, SVP) A parenteral drug is defined as one intended for injection through the skin or other external boundary tissue, rather than through the alimentary canal, so that active substances they contain are administered, using gravity or force, directly into a blood vessel, organ, tissue, or lesion. It is infused when administered intravenously (IV), or injected when administered intramuscularly (IM), or subcutaneously into the human body. A large volume parenteral (LVP) is a unit dose container of greater than 100 ml that is terminally sterilized by heat and small volume parenteral (SVP) is a catch-all for all non-LVP parenteral products except biologicals.

Parenteral route A route of drug administration, which is non-oral, e.g. by injection.

Paresthesia A sensation of numbness, prickling, or tingling of the skin.

Parfocal A microscope, which retains proper focus when the objectives are changed.

Parietal When the placenta is attached to the wall of the ovary.

Parietal cell Of ovule, development, referring to the cell(s) cut off from the archesporial cell(s) prior to meiosis and forming part of the nucellus (in the ovule) and the endothecium (in the anther).

Paronychia Inflammation involving the folds of tissue surrounding the nail, which is usually caused by *Candida albicans*.

Parthenocarpy Development of fruit without fertilization and seed.

Parthenogenesis Development of an egg without fertilization.

Partial agonist A partial agonist is an agonist that is unable to induce maximal activation of a receptor population, regardless of the amount of drug applied.

Partial pressure Refers to the pressure exerted by a certain gas in a mixture.

Particle Small portion of matter.

Particle concentration Number of individual particles per unit volume of air.

Partition coefficient The partition coefficient of a drug is the ratio of the solubility of the drug, at equilibrium, in a nonaqueous solvent, (e.g. b-octanol) to that in an aqueous solvent, (e.g. water; pH 7.4, buffer solution).

Parturient A substance, which induces and promotes labor.

Parturifacient Herbs or substances that induces child-birth or labor.

Passage cells Cells of the endodermis opposite the protoxylem, which remain thin-walled and retain their Casparian band, or a similar cell in the exodermis.

Passivation A final chemical treatment/cleaning process, which removes exogenous iron or iron compounds from the surface of stainless steel piping and equipment by the use of a mild oxidant, such as a nitric acid solution, or by in situ electropoli-

shing. The intention of passivation is to restore and/or enhance the spontaneous formation of the chemically inert surface or protective passive film.

Passive diffusion The process in which molecules move from a region of higher concentration to one of lower concentration as a result of random thermal agitation.

Passive immunity Temporary immunity produced by administration of gamma globulin.

Passive transport Diffusion across a plasma membrane in which the cell expends no energy.

Passive vaccination Passive vaccination is the intramuscular or intravenous injection of antibody preparations to enhance a patient's immune competence.

Passivity The state in which a stainless steel exhibits a very low corrosion rate, also known as passivity, is the loss (or minimizing) of chemical reactivity exhibited by certain metals and alloys under particular environmental conditions.

Pasteur effect The decrease in the rate of sugar catabolism and change to aerobic respiration, which occurs when microorganisms are switched from anaerobic to aerobic conditions.

Pasteurization The heating of milk, wines, fruit juices, etc. for about thirty minutes at 68°C (154.4°F) whereby the living bacteria are destroyed, but the flavor or bouquet is preserved; the spores are unaffected, but are kept from developing by immediately cooling the liquid to 10°C (50°F) or lower.

Pathogen Refers to any microbiological or eukaryotic cell containing sufficient genetic information, which upon expression of such information is able of producing disease in healthy people, plants, or animals.

Pathogenic Causing or capable of causing disease.

Pathogenic organisms Organisms that are capable of causing disease, either directly (by infecting) or indirectly (by producing a toxin that causes illness).

Pathogenicity The condition or quality of being pathogenic, or the ability to cause disease.

p-coumaric acid A hydroxy acid derived from L:phenylalanine, involved in formation of phenylpropanoids, readily convertible into salicylic acid.

Pearl gland A small sessile spherical multicellular gland.

Pectin Refers to a highly hydrophilic polysaccharide built up of monomers of alpha-galacturonic acid, an important component of cell walls.

Pectinase An enzyme which is destroying the pectin of the middle lamella of cell-walls, produced by many parasitic fungi.

Pectinate Comb-like.

Pectoral Relieves disorders of the chest and lungs, such as an expectorant.

Ped A natural soil aggregate, formed partly through bacterial and fungal growth in the soil.

Pedicel The stalk of a flower in an inflorescence.

Pedigree analysis Refers to a type of genetic analysis in which a trait is traced through several generations of a family inorder to determine how the trait is inherited.

Peduncle The stem of an individual flower or fruit.

Peg roots Primary roots.

Pelagic Living in the open ocean, offshore.

Pelargonidin An anthocyanin.

Pellicle A relatively rigid layer of proteinaceous elements, which is just beneath the plasma membrane in many protozoa and algae. The plasma membrane is sometimes considered as a part of the pellicle. For plants, the covering (skin), which encloses the kernel; it is white during development but becomes brown at maturity.

Pellucid Transparent.

Peltate Leaves, which are shaped like a shield and attached to the stem at the center or by some point distinctly within the margin, and having the petiole inserted into the undersurface of the lamina not far from the center.

Pelvic inflammatory disease (PID) A severe infection of the female reproductive organs, the disease that results when gonococci and chlamydiae infect the uterine tubes and surrounding tissue.

Pelvis Refers to the hollow cavity formed by the two hipbones.

Pendulous Drooping, of ovules, especially those attached at or near the apex of the loculus and so borne pendulous on an apical placenta.

Penetrance A term indicating the likelihood that a given gene will actually result in disease.

Penicillin An antibiotic containing a ß-lactam ring that inhibits an enzyme responsible for making peptide cross-links in the bacterial cell wall, obtained from cultures of the molds *Penicillium notatum* or *Penicillium chrysogenum*.

Penicillium The genus of mold causing a zone of inhibition in an agar plate of bacteria, it produces natural penicillin.

Peniculiate With the form of a pencil.

Penninerved Pinnate venation.

Penton or pentamer A capsomer composed of five protomers.

Pentose Refers to any of the 5-carbon sugars e.g., ribose, deoxy ribose, xylose and arabinose that are synthesized from hexoses in pentose phosphate pathway from CO_2 in calvin cycle or by decarboxylation of nucleic diphosphate sugars.

Pentose phosphate pathway The pathway, which oxidizes glucose 6-phosphate to ribulose 5-phosphate and then converts it to a variety of three to seven carbon sugars; it forms several important products (NADPH for biosynthesis, pentoses, and other sugars) and also can be used to degrade glucose to CO_2.

Peplomer or spike A protein or protein complex, which extends from the virus envelope and often is important in virion attachment to the host cell surface.

Pepsi An enzyme produced from pepsinogen, which initiates protein digestion by breaking down protein into large peptide fragments, or an enzyme, produced by the stomach, that chemically breaks down peptide bonds in polypeptides and proteins.

Pepsinogen An inactive form of pepsin, synthesized and stored in cells lining the gastric pits of the stomach.

Peptic An herb or substance that aides in the digestion of food.

Peptic ulcer disease A gastritis caused by *Helicobacter pylori*.

Peptide A secondary protein derivative defined as a definitely characterized combination of two or more amino acids, the carboxyl (COOH) group of one being united with the amino (NH_2) group of the other, with the elimination of a molecule of water. They form a peptide bond or short chains of amino acids.

Peptide bond A covalent bond, which links two amino acids together to form a polypeptide chain.

Peptide hormones A diverse class of hormones, which are synthesized and excreted at various sites within the body, e.g. insulin, relaxin, glucagons, growth hormone, vasopressin, ACTH (adrenocorticotropic hormone), endorphins, and encephalins.

Peptide interbridge A short peptide chain, which connects the tetrapeptide chains in some peptidoglycans.

Peptidoglycan Refers to a large polymer composed of long chains of alternating N-acetylglucosamine and N-acetylmuramic acid residues. The polysaccharide chains are linked to each other through connections between tetrapeptide chains attached to the N-acetylmuramic acids. It provides much of the strength and rigidity for the bacterial cell walls.

Peptidomimetic A peptidomimetic is a compound containing non-peptidic structural elements, which is capable of mimicking or antagonizing the biological action(s) of a natural parent peptide. It no longer have classical peptide characteristics such as enzymatically scissille peptidic bonds.

Peptidyl or donor site (P site) The site on the ribosome, which contains the peptidyl-tRNA at the beginning of the elongation cycle during protein synthesis.

Peptidyl transferase The enzyme, which catalyzes the transpeptidation reaction in protein synthesis; in this reaction, an amino acid is added to the growing peptide chain.

Peptoid A peptoid is a peptidomimetic, which results from the oligomeric assembly of N-substituted glycines.

Peptones They are water-soluble digests or hydrolysates of proteins, which are used in the preparation of culture media.

Percent composition Expresses the weight ratio between different elements in a compound.

Percentage volume-in-volume (v/v) Percentage v/v indicates the number of milliliters of a constant in 100 ml of liquid formulation.

Percentage weight-in-volume (w/v) Percentage w/v indicates the number of grams of a constituent per 100 ml of solution or liquid formulation.

Percentage weight-in-weight (w/w) Percent w/w indicates the number of grams of a constant per 100 g of formulation (solid or liquid).

Percolation A process to extract the soluble constituents of a plant with the assistance of gravity. The material is moistened and evenly packed into a tall, slightly conical vessel; the liquid (menstruum) is then poured on to the material and allowed to steep for a certain length of time. A small opening is then made in the bottom, which allows the extract to slowly flow out of the vessel. The remaining plant material (the marc) may be discarded. Many tinctures and liquid extracts are prepared this way.

Perennating Maintaining a dormant, vegetative state throughout the non-growing seasons.

Perennation Survival of a plant for a number of years, to live over from season to season.

Perennial A plant, which grows for 3 or more years and usually flowers each year.

Perfect flower A flower with both essential and accessory organs.

Perfoliate Refers to opposite or whorled leaves or bracts that are united into a collar-like structure around the stem that bears them.

Perforation plate Refers to a vessel in particular, the end wall between vessel elements that is variously broken down.

Perforin pathway The cytotoxic pathway that uses perforin protein, which polymerizes to form membrane pores that help destroy cells during cell-mediated cytotoxicity. Perforin is produced by cytotoxic T cells and NK cells and stored in granules, which are released when a target cell is contacted.

Peri (prefix) Surrounding.

Perianth The outer whorl of floral leaves of a flower, when not clearly divided into calyx and corolla; collectively, the calyx and corolla, or either one if one is absent.

Periblem Term used for the middle of the three histogen layers that were supposed to make up the apical meristem, giving rise to the cortex.

Pericarp The fruit wall which has developed from the ovary wall; sometimes used for any fruit covering.

Pericarpium Refers to the peel or rind of fruit.

Periclinal Those parallel to the surface.

Pericycle The outermost part of the stele, often parenchymatous, but fibers and/or sclereids are often also found in this general area. The layer between endodermis and conducting tissues.

Pericyclic fibres Fibres in the pericycle.

Periderm Several layers of corky cells located on the outside of the epidermis and containing high amounts of suberin.

Perigenous Refers to stomatal ontogeny in which the subsidiary cells are not produced from the same cell (meristemoid, initial) that gives rise to the guard cell initials.

Perigonium A collective term used to refer to the two whorls of an undifferentiated perianth when these cannot be distinguished.

Period of infectivity Refers to the time during which the source of an infectious disease is infectious or is disseminating the pathogen.

Periodic table Grouping of the known elements by their number of protons. There are many other trends such as size of elements and electronegativity, which are easily expressed in terms of the periodic table.

Periodontal disease A disease located around the teeth or in the periodontium—the tissue investing and supporting the teeth, including the cementum, periodontal ligament, alveolar bone, and gingiva.

Periodontosis A degenerative, noninflammatory condition of the periodontium that is characterized by destruction of tissue.

Peripheral nervous system The division of the nervous system, which connects the central nervous system to other parts of the body.

Periplasm The substance that fills the periplasmic space.

Periplasmic flagella The flagella, which lie under the outer sheath and extend from both ends of the spirochete cell to overlap in the middle and form the axial filament. Also called axial fibrils and endoflagella.

Periplasmic space or periplasm Refers to the fluid occupying the space between the inside and outside cellular membranes of bacteria.

Perisperm Diploid nutritive tissue in an angiospermous seed, derived from nucellar tissue.

Peristalsis Involuntary contractions of the smooth muscles in the walls of the esophagus, stomach, and intestines, which propel food along the digestive tract.

Peristaltic pump A type of positive displacement pump, which operates by pulsations of flow caused by passing rollers over flexible tubing. Operating pressure limited by tubing tolerance.

Peristome A set of cells or cell parts, which enclose the opening of a moss sporangium. In many mosses, they are sensitive to humidity, and will alter their shape to help in spore dispersal.

Perithecium A globular to flask-shaped fruiting body that has an apical pore through which the spores (ascospores) are released.

Peritrichous A cell with flagella evenly distributed over its surface.

Permeability The ability of a body to pass a fluid under pressure.

Permease A membrane-bound carrier protein or a system of two or more proteins, which transports a substance across the membrane.

Peroxidase An enzyme that catalyzes the oxidation of a substrate by the removal of hydrogen. The hydrogen is removed by its combination with hydrogen peroxide.

Peroxisome Very small membrane-bound particles responsible for photorespiration in plants, similar to lysosome in structure, but not in function, or membrane-bound vesicles in eukaryotic cells that contain oxidative enzymes.

Persistent Remaining attached after the normal function has been completed.

Persistent virus A virus, which systemically infects its insect vector and usually is transmitted for the remainder of the vector's life.

Pertussis An acute, highly contagious infection of the respiratory tract, most frequently affecting young children, usually caused by *Bordetella pertussis* or *B. parapertussis*. It consists of peculiar paroxysms of coughing, ending in a prolonged crowing or whooping respiration, so the name whooping cough.

Pessary It is a small plastic or silicone medical device or form of pharmaceutical preparation that is inserted into the vagina or rectum and held in place by the pelvic floor musculature.

Pest Refers to any organism, which damages and reduces the crop or irritates or injures live stock.

Pest resurgence The rapid rebound of a pest population after it has been controlled.

Pesticide resistance The genetically acquired ability of an organism to survive a pesticide application at doses that once killed most individuals of the same species.

Pesticide Any substance or mixture intended for preventing, destroying, repelling, killing, or mitigating problems caused by any insects, rodents, weeds, nematodes, fungi, or other pests; and any other substance or mixture intended for use as a plant growth regulator, defoliant, or desiccant.

Pet therapy A therapeutic approach based on the idea that expressing affection for a pet helps people feel happier, maintain a positive outlook, and therefore improve their health. According to several studies, having a pet can reduce stress, lower blood pressure, and ward off loneliness and depression. Many nursing homes and some prisons have developed pet therapy programs, with excellent results.

Petal Any of the component parts, or leaves, of a corolla; the unit of structure of the corolla.

Petaloid Like a petal.

Petiolate Growing on, or provided with, a petiole.

Petiole The slender stalk or stem of a leaf, also called a leaf stalk.

Petri dish A shallow dish consisting of two round, overlapping halves that is used to grow microorganisms on solid culture medium. The top lid is larger than the bottom of the dish to prevent contamination of the culture.

Petrifaction Mode of fossilization where the organic matter is replaced with silica.

Petrolatum White petrolatum is a purified mixture of semi-solid hydrocarbons, which is obtained from petroleum, common base or carrier for ointments.

Petroselinic acid A mono-unsaturated fatty acid with the double bond in the delta-6 position.

pH The pH value of an aqueous solution is a number describing its acidity or alkalinity. A pH is the negative logarithm (base 10) of the concentration of hydrogen ions (equivalent per liter). The pH value of a neutral solution is 7. An acidic solution has a pH less than 7, while a basic solution has a pH greater than 7, up to 14.

Phage Refers to a virus for which the natural host is a bacterial cell.

Phagocyte A cell, which engulfs foreign particles from its surroundings by a process called phagocytosis. The cell releases hydrolytic enzymes from intracellular bodies called lysosomes, which partially digest the foreign particle, after which it is further degraded in the phagocyte cytoplasm.

Phagocytic vacuole A membrane-delimited vacuole produced by cells carrying out phagocytosis. It is formed by the invagination of the plasma membrane and contains solid material.

Phagocytosis Refers to the endocytotic process in which a cell encloses large particles in a membrane-delimited phagocytic vacuole or phagosome and engulfs them.

Phagolysosome The vacuole, which results from the fusion of a phagosome with a lysosome.

Phagotrophy Endocytosis or engulfing particles of food as a mode of nutrition.

Phagovar A specific phage type.

Phanerogam A plant with conspicuous reproductive parts, a plant with seeds as its main dispersal units.

Phanerophyte Refers to life forms, plants with resting buds 25 cm or more above the surface of the ground.

Pharmaceutical A medicinal drug, or relating to or engaged in pharmacy or the manufacture and sale of pharmaceuticals. A pharmaceutical product is generally one, which is made up using available chemical compounds.

Pharmaceutical alternatives Pharmaceutical alternatives are drug products that contain the same therapeutic moiety but are different salts, esters, or complexes (e.g. tetracycline hydrochloride versus tetracycline phosphate); or are different dosage forms (e.g. tablet versus capsule; immediate release dosage form versus controlled release dosage form); or strengths.

Pharmaceutical equivalents Pharmaceutical equivalents are drug products that contain the same therapeutically active drug ingredient(s), same salt, ester, or chemical form; are of the same dosage form; and are identical in strength and concentration and route of administration. Pharmaceutical equivalents may differ in characteristics such as shape, scoring configuration, release mechanisms, packaging, and excipients (including colors, flavoring, preservatives).

Pharmaceutical principles Pharmaceutical principles are the underlying physicochemical principles that allow a drug to be incorporated in a pharmaceutical dosage form (e.g. solution, capsule). These principles apply whether the drug is extemporaneously compounded by the pharmacist or manufactured for commercial distribution as a drug product.

Pharmaceutics It is the discipline of pharmacy which deals with all facets of the process of turning a new chemical entity (NCE) into a medication able to be safely and effectively used by patients in the community. Pharmaceutics is the science of dosage form design.

Pharmacodynamics The study of the physiological effects and mechanisms of action of a compound and how this varies with concentration/dosage, or, the study of how the drug acts upon the body.

Pharmacognosy The study of natural products (i.e. plant, animal, organism, or mineral in nature) used as drugs or for the preparation of drugs, word derived from the Greek *Pharmakon* meaning drug and *Gnosis* meaning knowledge.

Pharmacokinetic dosing Dosing a drug based on blood levels and the ability to eliminate the drug from the body with the goal of attaining efficacious blood levels while avoiding toxicity.

Pharmacokinetics The study of how compounds are absorbed, distributed, metabolized and eliminated by the body, or, the study of how the body acts upon the drug.

Pharmacovigilance The constant monitoring of the safe use of medicinal products. Pharmacovigilance is generally regarded as all post-authorisation scientific and data-gathering activities aimed at detecting, assessing, understanding, and preventing adverse events or reactions or any other problems related to the use of a pharmaceutical product. This enables an ongoing assessment to make sure that only those medicines presenting a positive benefit-to-risk ratio remain in use.

Pharmacy-compounding An old fashion type of pharmacy that still mixes medications to doctors orders such as pouring prescribed amounts of a drug powder into capsules.

Pharynx Refers to the passage way between the mouth and the esophagus and trachea.

Phase-contrast microscope A microscope, which converts slight differences in refractive index and cell density into easily observed differences in light intensity.

Phase inversion Phase inversion, or emulsion-type reversal, involves the reversion of an emulsion from an oil in water (o/w) to a water in oil (w/o) form, or vice versa. Phase inversion can change the consistency or texture of the emulsion or cause further deterioration in its stability.

Phaseollin A phytoalexin, kind of isoflavonoid.

Phellem Cork.

Phelloderm Tissue derived from the activity of the cork cambium, the cells being parenchymatous (usually) and cut off internally.

Phellogen Cork cambium.

Phenetic system A classification system, which groups organisms together based on the similarity of their observable characteristics.

Phenol An acidic aromatic compound, a common constituent of organic compounds such as cinnamic acid.

Phenol coefficient test A test to measure the effectiveness of disinfectants by comparing their activity against test bacteria with that of phenol.

Phenol red Phenolsulfonphthalein, $C_{19}H_{14}O_5S$, an acid-base indicator that changes from yellow to red as the pH passes through 8.

Phenolic A molecule containing an aromatic ring, which bears one or more hydroxyl groups is referred to as 'phenolic.' Examples include flavonoids, isoflavonoids, etc.

Phenotype The characters of an organism due to the interaction of genotype and environment, a group of individuals exhibiting the same phenotypic characters. The detectable expression of the interaction of genotype and environment constituting the visible characters of an organism.

Phenotypic A set of characters arising from reaction to environmental stimulus.

Phenoxy herbicides Refer to a group of herbicides derived from phenoxy-acetic acid, including 2,4-D, 2,4,5-T, 2,4-DB, MCPA and silvex.

Phenylphenalenones Group of phytoalexins, in this remove the phenyl group to the right and you have phenalenone.

Phenylpropanoids Any compound bearing a 3-carbon chain attached to a 6-carbon aromatic ring (C6-C3 compounds), most being formed from cinnamic or p-coumaric acids, volatile compounds in essential oils.

Pheromone A substance secreted by an organism to affect the behavior or development of other members of the same species, sex pheromones, which attract the opposite sex for mating are used in monitoring certain insects.

Pherophyll A foliage leaf or bract subtending an axillary shoot or flower.

Phlobaphene A brownish material perhaps related to proanthocyanidins or non-hydrolyzable tannins and found, e.g. in the testa of some seeds.

Phloem The tissue involved in the transport of carbohydrates and food materials in a vascular plant, being composed of sieve elements, parenchyma cells and sometimes also of fibers and sclereids.

Phlogistic Refers to inflammation or fever.

Phloroglucinol Simple phenolic compound that is composed of an aromatic ring and three hydroxyl groups, an aglycone of many glycosides.

Phosphatase An enzyme, which catalyzes the hydrolytic removal of phosphate from molecules.

Phosphate group A chemical group, which is composed of a central phosphorus bonded to three or four oxygens.

Phosphate group transfer potential A measure of the ability of a phosphorylated molecule like ATP to transfer its phosphate to water and other acceptors.

Phospholipids Lipids with a phosphate group in place of one of the three fatty acid chains, asymmetrical molecules with a hydrophilic head and a hydrophobic tail. They are the building blocks of cellular membranes.

Phosphorylation A process that involves the transfer of a phosphate group (catalyzed by enzymes) from a donor to a suitable acceptor.

Photic zone The layer of the ocean, which is penetrated by sunlight that extends to a depth of about 200 meters.

Photoautotrophs Facultative autotrophs, which obtain their energy from light.

Photolithotrophic autotrophs Organisms, which use light energy, an inorganic electron source, (e.g. H_2O, H_2, H_2S), and CO_2 as a carbon source.

Photoluminescent The property of emitting light as the result of absorption of visible or invisible light that continues for a length of time after excitation.

Photo-organotrophic heterotrophs Microorganisms, which use light energy and organic electron donors, and also employ simple organic molecules rather than CO_2 as their carbon source.

Photolysis The cleavage of one or more covalent bonds in a molecular entity that results from absorption of light, or a photochemical process in which such cleavage is an essential part.

Photons Massless packet of energy that behaves like both a wave and a particle.

Photo-oxidation The mechanism by which ultraviolet light reduces total organic carbon (TOC) to carbon dioxide. If halogenated organics are present, both CO_2 and mineral acids can be formed.

Photoperiodism The response of a plant to periods of light and darkness, particularly as regards the beginning of flowering.

Photosensitivity Abnormal sensitivity to sunlight or artificial forms of ultraviolet radiation, like the one emitted from fluorescent light tubes.

Photosynthate The products of photosynthesis, used to support growth, respiration, and fruit production.

Photosynthesis Refers to the sequence of events taking place in green plants and photosynthetic bacteria in which light energy of solar radition gets traped and converted into chemical energy of bonds in complex organic carbohydrates that are synthesized by involving inorganic substances like CO_2 and water and concomitant release of oxygen. In other words the process by which plants convert sunlight into energy.

Photosystem A membrane-bound protein complex in plants and photosynthetic bacteria, responsible for light harvesting and primary electron transfer. Comprises light-harvesting pigments such as chlorophyll; a primary electron-transfer center, and secondary electron carriers.

Phototropism The directional growth response (tropism) of a plant or part of a plant to light.

Phototrophs Organisms, which use light as their energy source.

Phragmoplast Microfibrils, which are parallel to the spindle axis at telophase across which a cell plate is deposited in cell division.

Phycobilin Biliprotein pigments.

Phycobiliproteins Photosynthetic pigments that are composed of proteins with attached tetrapyrroles, they are often found in cyanobacteria and red algae.

Phycobilisomes Special particles on the membranes of cyanobacteria, which contain photosynthetic pigments and electron transport chains.

Phycobiont The algal or cyanobacterial partner in a lichen.

Phycocyanin A blue phycobiliprotein pigment that is used to trap light energy during photosynthesis.

Phycoerythrin A red photosynthetic phycobiliprotein pigment that is used to trap light energy.

Phycology The study of algae, algology.

Phycomycetes Alga-like fungi, which do not possess chlorophyll and cannot photosynthesize. Aquatic and terrestrial molds belong to this category.

Phycoplast Assemblage of microtubules perpendicular to the spindle and at the equator of the cell at telophase in cell division.

Phyliary Inflorescence bract of an involucre, as in asteraceae.

Phylloclade A flattened, more or less leaf-like, photosynthetic stem of a plant whose photosynthetic leaves are much reduced.

Phyllode A leaf whose blade is much reduced or absent, and whose petiole and/or rachis have assumed the functions of the whole leaf.

Phyllome A collective term for all the leaf structures of a plant.

Phyllosphere The surface of plant leaves.

Phyllosporous Refers to sporangia borne on a leaf.

Phyllotaxy The arrangement of the leaves on the stem.

Phylogenetic or phyletic classification system A classification system based on evolutionary relationships rather than the general similarity of contemporary characteristics.

Phylogenetic tree A graph made of nodes and branches, much like a tree in shape, that shows phylogenetic relationships between groups of organisms and sometimes also indicates the evolutionary development of groups.

Phylogeny The racial history or evolutionary development of any plant or animal species.

Phylum Primary taxonomic grouping, division.

Physical hazard A classification of a chemical for which there is scientifically valid evidence that it is a combustible liquid, compressed gas, cryogenic, explosive, flammable gas, flammable liquid, flammable solid, organic peroxide, oxidizer, pyrophoric, unstable, reactive, or water-reactive material.

Physical property A property, which can be measured without changing the chemical composition of a substance.

Physical therapy Therapy, which assists patients in improving their ability to move, reducing pain, and regain posture and balance.

Physiological concentrations Concentrations of a substance likely to occur within the human body.

Physiological disorder A disorder caused by factors other than a pathogen, abiotic disorder.

Phytoalexin An antimicrobial, protective compound synthesized by a plant in response to bacterial, viral, or fungal infection, many chemicals, which are medicinal to humans are phytoalexins.

Phytochelatin A peptide of higher plants, consisting of polymers of 2-11 glutathione (γ-glutamyl-cysteinyl-glycine) groups that binds heavy metals.

Phytochemicals Chemical compounds or chemical constituents formed in the plant's normal metabolic processes. The chemicals are often referred to as "secondary metabolites" of which there are several classes including alkaloids, anthraquinones, coumarins, fats, flavonoids, glycosides, gums, iridoids, mucilages, phenols, phytoestrogens, tannins, terpenes, and terpenoids, to mention a few. Extracts contain many chemical constituents, while chemicals that have been isolated from the plant are considered pharmaceutical drugs, (i.e. atropine, digoxin, morphine, etc.).

Phytochemistry The branch of chemistry, which focuses on the constituents of plants (phyto comes from the Greek word for plant). Often, phytochemistry deals specifically with the chemistry of medicinal plants. This discipline can also include studies of how to extract, concentrate, analyze, standardize, and preserve herbal products.

Phytochrome A pigment in plant leaves, which detects day length and generates a response and is partly responsible for photoperiodism.

Phytoestrogens A type of phytochemical with some influence on the estrogenic activity or hormonal system in humans, does not mean that the plant mimics human estrogen, only acts to affect it in some way.

Phytoferritin An iron-protein complex, present as crystalline inclusions in some plastids.

Phytohormone A substance that is produced by plants, which influence the growth and/or develop all part of the plant.

Phytomedicinals Medicinal substances, which originate from plants. This may include certain phytochemicals as well as whole plants or herbal preparations.

Phytomelan Black, carbonaceous material forming a crust-like covering of some seeds.

Phytoplankton A community of floating photosynthetic organisms, mainly composed of algae and cyanobacteria.

Phytoremediation The use of plants and their associated microorganisms to remove, contain, or degrade environmental contaminants.

Phytosomes They are advanced forms of herbal products that are better absorbed, utilized, and as a result produce better results than conventional herbal extracts. They are produced via a patented process whereby the individual components of an herbal extract are bound to phosphatidylcholine—an emulsifying compound derived from soy.

Phytotoxicity The ability of a material such as a pesticide or fertilizer to cause injury to plants.

Pi bonds A type of covalent bond in which the electron density is concentrated around the line bonding the atoms.

Picket-fence porphyrin A porphyrin with a protective enclosure for binding oxygen at one side of the ring, which is used to mimic the dioxygen-carrying properties of the heme group.

Picking Picking is removal of the surface material of a tablet by a punch.

Piedra A fungal disease of the hair in which white or black nodules of fungi form on the shafts.

Pileus Umbrella-shaped structure of mushrooms or toadstools.

Pili Pili (imbriae) are protienaceous hairs that are shorter than flagella, composed of regularly arranged protein subunits and are called pilin or fimbrilin. They are more common in gram-negative organisms but can be found in gram-positive organisms.

Pilose Hairy, pubescence comprised of scattered long, slender, soft hairs.

Pinnate Divided in a feathery manner, with lateral processes of a compound leaf, having leaflets on each side of an axis or midrib.

Pinnately compound Leaves that are divided up like a feather are said to be pinnately compound.

Pinnatifid Refers to leaf, cut about half the width of the leaf blade into lobes that are spaced out along the midrib.

Pinnatinerved Refers to venation, pinnate.

Pinnatipartite Refers to leaves with lobing over two-thirds of the distance to the midrib, but the parenchyma is not interrupted.

Pinnatisect Refers to leaf blade, dissected down to the midrib, the parenchyma being interrupted.

Pinocytosis The endocytotic process in which a cell encloses a small amount of the surrounding liquid and its solutes in tiny pinocytotic vesicles or pinosomes.

Pioneer species A plant species, which colonizes habitat that was previously unoccupied or sparsely occupied by that species. In the successive settlement of an area by plant species, such as after a fire, pioneer species lead the process.

Piperidine alkaloids A group of alkaloids whose structure is based on piperidine ring, most are derived from amino acid lysine, e.g. nicotine.

Pistil The unit of female function of a flower, may be comprised of a single carpel or two or more carpels united.

Pistillate Refers to a flower bearing a pistil or pistils but not stamens, may refer also to a plant having only pistillate flowers.

Pit Any interruption in the secondary cell wall, pits in the xylem may be bordered, scalariform, simple or vestured, and borne in an alternate or opposite arrangement.

Pitched Pertains to inoculation of a nutrient medium with yeast, e.g. in beer brewing.

Pith The central region of a stem, the inner part of the stele that is produced by differentiation of the ground meristem.

Pits Thin regions of the cell wall in xylem conducting cells. Their structure is an important characteristic for recognizing different kinds of wood.

Placebo A pharmacologically inactive substance, primarily used in experiments to provide a basis for comparison with pharmacologically active substances.

Placenta The part of the ovary from which the ovules arise, generally occupies the whole or a portion of an angle of a cell.

Placentation The manner in which the placenta is arranged in the ovary.

Plagiotropic A gravitational response that results in the stem being held more or less horizontal.

Plague An acute febrile, infectious disease, caused by the bacillus *Yersinia pestis* that has a high mortality rate; the two major types are bubonic plague and pneumonic plague.

Planate Flat.

Plankton Free-floating, mostly microscopic microorganisms, which can be found in almost all waters; a collective name (or) drifting organisms.

Plano-convex Flat on one side and convex on the other.

Planozygote A motile zygote.

Plant Any of a kingdom (Plantae) of living beings typically lacking locomotive movement or obvious sensory organs, generally making its own food, possessing cell walls, and unlimited growth.

Plantlet A little plant. Plants reproducing by spores and not seeds, e.g. ferns, mosses, fungi, etc.

Plaque A scar created by areas of demyelination or inflammation in the central nervous system tissue.

Plasma The liquid portion of blood in which the cellular elements are suspended, a fresh liquid obtained by centrifugation, plasma is a clear, amber-colored solution containing 8 to 9% solids; among these, 85% are proteins while the other components are the lipids, which include the neutral fats, fatty acids, lecithin, and cholesterol. Also sodium, chloride and bicarbonate, potassium, calcium and magnesium are presnt. A most vital function of plasma is the maintenance of blood pressure and the exchange with tissue of nutrients for waste.

Plasma cell A mature, differentiated B lymphocyte chiefly occupied with antibody synthesis and secretion, lives for only 5 to 7 days.

Plasma membrane The selectively permeable membrane surrounding the cell's cytoplasm, also called the cell membrane, plasmalemma, or cytoplasmic membrane.

Plasmid A double-stranded DNA molecule, which can exist and replicate independently of the chromosome or may be integrated with it. A plasmid is stably inherited, but is not required for the host cell's growth and reproduction.

Plasmid fingerprinting A technique used to identify microbial isolates as belonging to the same strain because they contain the same number of plasmids with the identical molecular weights and similar phenotypes.

Plasmodesmata Refers to cytoplasmic connections between neighboring cells in plant tissues.

Plasmodial (acellular) slime mold A member of the division Myxomycota, which exists as a thin, streaming, multinucleate mass of protoplasm that creeps along in an amoeboid fashion.

Plasmodium Refers to a stage in the life cycle of myxomycetes (plasmodial slime molds); a multinucleate mass of protoplasm surrounded by a membrane. Also, refers to a parasite of the genus Plasmodium.

Plasmolysis The process in which water osmotically leaves a cell that causes the cytoplasm to shrivel up and pull the plasma membrane away from the cell wall.

Plastics High molecular weight polymers or copolymers.

Plasticity It is the ability of the plants to adapt to environmental conditions by altering their metabolism, growth and development inorder to suit their environment.

Plastid A cytoplasmic organelle of algae and higher plants, which contains pigments such as chlorophyll, stores food reserves, and often carries out processes such as photosynthesis.

Plastochrone Time interval between two successive events, like initiation of leaf primordia.

Platyspermic With seeds which are flattened and disc-like.

Plectostele Refers to a variant of a protostele in which the xylem and phloem form more or less parallel bands.

Pleomorphic Refers to bacteria that are variable in shape and lack a single, characteristic form.

Plena The plural of plenum.

Plenum An enclosure in which air or other gas is at a pressure greater than that outside the enclosure.

Pleura A thin sheet of epithelium, which covers the inside of the thoracic cavity and the outer surface of the lungs.

Plicate Folded like a paper fan, as in the leaves of palms, cyclanthoids, and some orchids.

Plumbagin A naphthoquinone derived from six C2 units, the acetate arising from L-tyrosine as opposed to the typical derivation from the shikimic acid pathway.

Plumbum Latin for lead, so the symbol Pb.

Plumose With hair-like branches, feathery.

Plumule The young shoot above the cotyledon(s)of an embryo or seedling.

Plurilocular With many small chambers or locules.

Pneumatophore An aertaing organ, often containing aerenchyma, which project above the level of the water.

Pneumonia Disease with many varieties characterized mainly by inflammation of the lungs and the symptoms include chest pain, cough, phlegm, aches, and fever.

Pocosin A bog, which has formed in a shallow, undrained depression, the surrounding land being somewhat elevated, the vegetation predominantly evergreen shrubs or small trees. They vary greatly in size.

Pod Often used for the fruit of any member of Fabaceae (Leguminaceae), since it can be fleshy, dry, winged or not, dehiscent, indehiscent, etc.

Point mutation A mutation, which affects only a single base pair in a specific location.

Poison Any substance which when taken into the body in a single dose of 1.0 gm or less, is injurious to health or dangerous to life.

Polar Polar molecules are asymmetric and have nonzero dipole moments.

Polar covalent bond A covalent bond in that the atoms share electrons in an unequal fashion, resulting molecule has regions with positive and negative charges.

Polar flagellum A flagellum that is located at one end of an elongated cell.

Polar molecules Refer to the molecules with a partial charge.

Polarity Refers to the condition resulting from the establishment of definite orientation during differentiation as in cell tissue or organ. It is important in early growth of plants as is revealed by separate development of root and shoot system from initially formed bipolar embryo.

Poliomyelitis An acute, contagious viral disease, which attacks the central nervous system, injuring or destroying the nerve cells that control the muscles and sometimes causing paralysis; also called polio or infantile paralysis.

Polished water Refers to high purity water after it has undergone a second treatment step. Ultrapure water usually undergoes two or more treatment steps. More economical pretreatment

processes, (e.g. reverse osmosis) are used to remove all but a very small fraction of the impurities. Highly efficient polishing processes, (e. g. mixed-bed deionization) are used to remove the impurities that remain.

Pollen grain The microspore of seed plants.

Pollen kitt Material or fluid from the tapetum covering the pollen grains, sometimes causing them to stick together.

Pollen tube In seed plants, the extension of the male gametophyte as it emerges from the pollen grain in search of the female gametophyte.

Pollen The male or fertilizing element of seed plants that consists of fine yellowish powder formed within the anther of the stamen (microspore).

Pollination Process of transferring the pollen from its place of production to the place where the egg cell is produced, which may be accomplished by the use of wind, water, insects, birds, bats, or other means. Pollination is generally followed by fertilization, in which sperm are released from the pollen grain to unite with the egg cell.

Pollinator The agent of pollen transfer, generally bees.

Pollinizer The producer of pollen, the variety used as a source of pollen for cross-pollination.

Poly (prefix), Many, especially over 15 or so, or separate.

Polyacetylenes Unsaturated compounds derived from oleic acid by dehydrogenation, highly reactive but with additional functional groups such as alcohols, ketones, acids, esters, furans, or pyrans that tend to stabilize the reactive acetylenic bonds.

Polyad Refers to pollen aggregated into units of many grains each.

Polyderm Arises from a lateral meristem that develops in ground tissues located in the pericycle and which cuts off lamellae of paired concentric layers of parenchymatous and endodermal cells, externally.

Polyfructosans Fructose polysaccharides, e.g. inulin.

Polygamo-dioecious Polygamous but chiefly dioecious.

Polygamomonoecious With perfect, staminate and carpellate flowers on the same plant.

Polygamous Having bisexual, pistillate, and staminate flowers on the same individual plant.

Polygenic disorder Refers to a genetic disorder resulting from the combined action of alleles of more than one gene, (e.g. diabetes, and some cancers). Though such disorders are inherited, they depend on the simultaneous presence of several alleles and so the hereditary patterns are usually more complex than those of single gene disorders.

Polyglucan granules Polymers of glucose a bit like glycogen in animals.

Polyhydroxy alkaloids Indolizidine alkaloids, bicyclic alkaloids with fused 5- and 6-membered ring systems.

Polyhydroxylated A molecule bearing more than one hydroxyl group is called polyhydroxylated.

Polyisoprenes High molecular-weight terpenoids made up of many isoprene units, e.g. rubber.

Polyketides Compounds related to fatty acids composed of condensed acetate and malonate units with unreduced carbonyl units and aromatic ring systems, typically with phenolic substitutions.

Polymer A macromolecule (long chain) consisting of five or more repeating units called monomers, e.g. polyethylene, polystyrene, and PTFE (polytetrafluoroethylene).

Polymerase An enzyme, which catalyzes production of nucleic acid molecules.

Polymerase chain reaction (PCR) An in vitro technique that is used to synthesize large quantities of specific nucleotide sequences from small amounts of DNA. It employs oligonucleotide primers complementary to specific sequences in the target gene and special heat-stable DNA polymerases.

Polymerous Refers to parts of a flower, more than expected.

Polymorphic With more than two distinct morphological forms, either on a single plant or on different plants within a species.

Polymorphism Polymorphism is the condition wherein substances can exist in more than one crystalline form. These polymorphs have different molecular arrangements or crystal lattice structures. As a result, the different polymorphs of a drug solid can have different properties. For example, the melting point, solubility, dissolution rate, density, and stability can differ considerably among the polymorphic forms of a drug.

Polymorphonuclear leukocyte (PMN) A leukocyte, which has a variety of nuclear forms.

Polypeptide A long chain of amino acids covalently bound by peptide.

Polypetalous With many separate petals.

Polyphasic taxonomy An approach in which taxonomic schemes are developed using a wide range of phenotypic and genotypic information.

Polyribosome A complex of several ribosomes with a messenger RNA in which each ribosome translates the same message.

Polyploid With more than two of the basic haploid sets of chromosomes in the nucleus, represented as 3x, 4x, etc.

Polysaccharide A polymer made up of many hexose or pentose units, such as cellulose and glycogen, consist of long chains of monosaccharides.

Polysepalous With free sepals.

Polystromatic Blade of many cell layers.

Polysymmetric Symmetrical about more than two planes passing through the axis of the flower.

Polyxylic Seed plant stems with more than one vascular cylinder, each one with xylem and phloem.

Pome fruit A simple fleshy fruit, the outer portion of which is formed by the floral parts that surround the ovary.

Pond A body of standing water that is smaller than a lake, often artifically formed.

Population pharmacokinetics Population pharmacokinetics is the study of sources and correlates of variability in drug concentrations among individuals who are the target patient population. Population pharmacokinetics is most often applied to the clinical patient who is receiving relevant doses of a drug of interest. Both pharmacokinetic and non-pharmacokinetic data may be considered, including gender, age, weight, creatine clearance, and concomitant disease.

Porate A simple aperture in a pollen grain, which is more or less circular in surface view.

Porcine Relating to, or from swine (pigs) such as porcine growth hormone.

Pore A general term for any circular opening, thinner area, etc. through that the pollen escapes from an anther.

Poricidal Generally, opening by pores, of anthers.

Porin proteins Proteins, which form channels across the outer membrane of gram-negative bacterial cell walls. Small molecules are transported through these channels.

Porogamy Fertilisation during that the pollen tube penetrates the ovule by way of the micropyle.

Porphyrin A macrocyclic molecule that contains four pyrrole rings linked together by single carbon atom bridges between the alpha positions of the pyrrole rings. Porphyrins generally occur in their dianionic form coordinated to a metal ion.

Portal system An arrangement in that the capillaries drain into a vein, which opens into another capillary network.

Postemergence herbicide Refers to the herbicide applied after the emergence of weeds.

Postgenital Refers to fusion of parts, when parts that were initially free from one another grow together.

Postherpetic neuralgia The severe pain after a herpes infection.

Posttranscriptional modification The processing of the initial RNA transcript, heterogeneous nuclear RNA, to form mRNA.

Potable Suitable for drinking.

Potash Crude or purified potassium carbonate, K_2CO_3.

Potent A substance, which is active in relatively low doses or concentrations.

Potential energy The energy an object has because of its composition or position.

Potentized Generally refers to a substance prepared according to homeopathic pharmaceutical standards, which means that it has gone through serial dilution and succussion.

Poultice A therapeutic topical application of a soft moist mass of plant material (such as bruised fresh herbs), usually wrapped in a fine woven cloth.

Powders A pharmaceutical powder is a mixture of finely divided drugs or chemicals in dry form. The powder may be used internally or externally.

PPB (parts per billion) Parts per billion, or micrograms per liter.

PPM (parts per million) Abbreviation for parts per million, used to describe concentration in liquids or gases, e.g. 10,000 ppm is approximately equivalent to 10 g/ liter or a 1% W/V solution.

Pranayama A term from yoga and Ayurveda meaning breath control.

Prebiotics Food components, which escape digestion by normal human digestive enzymes and safely in intact form, reach the colon after passage through stomach and small intestine where they selectively promote the growth of probiotics, e.g. fructo-oligosaccharides, fructosan, etc.

Precipitate An insoluble reaction product. When a solution reaches saturation, solute will begin to come out of solution, as when water precipitates from the air as rain, or calcium carbonate precipitates out of water to form scale, the chalky white substance deposited on the inside of tea kettles.

Precommission Preparing the plant for commissioning (start-up), which includes briefly starting (bumping) all pieces of equipment, verifying their shaft rotation is correct, verifying that valves, gauges, and other inline devices are installed in the correct orientation, and performing functionality runs on all equipment and material, also includes leak tests.

Precursor Plants make phytochemicals by starting with one chemical, a parent compound, and changing it into another, called a derivative, meaning derived from the parent compound. Occurrence of chemical transformations where the original molecule changes shapes, splits up, or joins with other molecules or atoms on the way to becoming the derivative. Biochemists call this chain of transformative relationships a pathway. A pathway is organized by a specific group of enzymes, which help change each form of the molecule into the next form downstream. A molecule, which is upstream in this process is called a precursor of the final molecule.

Predator Any animal (including insects and mites) that kills other animals (prey) and feeds on them.

Predicate rules A previously published set of rules, like GLPs, GCP, or cGMPs, which mandate what records must be maintained, the required contents of those records, whether signatures are necessary, and how long the record must be maintained.

Preemergence herbicide Herbicide applied before emergence of weeds.

Prefilter A filter that is to trap gross particulates located upstream before an HEPA filter. The efficiency of initial prefilters is usually in the 20 to 30% range by the atmospheric dust spot efficiency, while intermediate prefilters usually have a collection efficiency of 80 to 90% by the same test.

Preformulation Preformulation is the characterization of the physical and chemical properties of the active drug substance and dosage form. The therapeutic indication of the drug and the route of administration will dictate the type of drug product or drug delivery system, (e.g. immediate release, controlled release, suppository, parenteral, transdermal) that needs to be developed.

Prenylation The attachment of a prenyl or isoprene unit, as in prenylated naphthoquinones.

Preservative A bacteriostatic or bacteriocidal agent added to preserve preparations, eg. benzalkonium chloride (BAC), formaldehyde, and thimerosol (merthiolate).

Pressure Force per unit area.

Pressure rating Pressure at which a system is designed to operate, allowing for applicable safety factors.

Prevalence rate Refers to the total number of individuals infected at any one time in a given population regardless of when the disease began.

Prickle Refers to a sharp pointed emergence arising from the epidermis or bark of a plant.

Primary air Air circulating through HEPA filters that is used to produce unidirectional flow in critical zones.

Primary bloom The first production of flowers on a potato plant that occurs when 8 to 12 leaves have been formed on the mainstem and generally coinciding with the beginning of the tuber growth phase.

Primary body Refers to those parts of a plant produced by the shoot and root apical meristems.

Primary compounds Chemicals that are made by plants and needed for their own metabolism.

Primary containment The first level of containment that consists of the inside portion of that container which comes into immediate contact on its inner surface with the material being contained.

Primary endosperm cell The cell formed by the fusion of the male gamete or sperm with the central cell of the embryo sac.

Primary growth Refers to the growth caused by the elongation and maturation of the primary tissues.

Primary inoculum The initial source of a pathogen, which starts disease development in a given location.

Primary leaf Refers to the first leaf of an embryo or seedling occurring above the cotyledonary node.

Primary macronutrients Refer to elements that plants require in relatively large quantities, like nitrogen, phosphorus, and potassium.

Primary meristem Apical meristem.

Primary metabolite A primary metabolite is essential for normal growth, development, and reproduction.

Primary producer Photoautotrophic and chemoautotrophic organisms, which incorporate carbon dioxide into organic carbon and thus provide new biomass for the ecosystem.

Primary production Refers to the incorporation of carbon dioxide into organic matter by photosynthetic organisms and chemoautotrophic bacteria.

Primary root Tap root.

Primary treatment Refers to the first step of sewage treatment, in which physical settling and screening are used to remove particulate materials.

Primary wall The first visible part of the cell wall deposited during extension growth of the cell and that is made up of cellulose fibrils, hemicelluloses, pectins, etc.

Primer Short pre-existing polynucleotide chain to which DNA polymerase can add new deoxyribonucleotides.

Primitive tannins Proanthocyanidins.

Primordium Organ of a plant as it first becomes apparent.

Prions Virus-like proteinaceous infectious agents, that differ from viruses in that they are not known to contain either DNA or RNA.

Proanthocyanidins Colorless glycosidic anthocyanidins, derived from isomerised flavonoids, usually polymers and based on monomeric flavan-3-ol (catechins) and flavan-3,4-diol units, also, colorless compounds that yield red anthocyanidins upon heating with acid.

Probiotics Microorganisms that when ingested with or without food improves the intestinal microbial balance and consequently the health and functioning of large intestine.

Procambium A primary meristem, which is near the apex of the stem or root and forming strands down the stem and root, differentiating to form primary vascular tissue.

Process aids Materials, excluding solvents that are used as an aid in the manufacture of an intermediate or API (active pharmaceutical ingredient) which themselves do not participate in a chemical or biological reaction, (e.g. filter aid, activated carbon, etc.).

Process suitability Refers to the established capacity of the manufacturing process to produce effective and reproducible results consistently.

Process validation Establishing, through documented evidence, a high degree of assurance, which a specific process will consistently produce a product that meets its predetermined specifications and quality characteristics.

Process validation protocol Documented plan for testing a pharmaceutical product and process to confirm that the production process used to manufacture the product performs as intended, includes a review of process variables and operational limitations as well as providing the sampling plan under actual use conditions.

Procumbent Trailing or lying flat but not rooting or trailing or spreading along the ground.

Prodrug A prodrug is any compound, which undergoes biotransformation before exhibiting its pharmacological effects. Prodrugs can thus be viewed as drugs containing specialized nontoxic protective groups used in a transient manner to alter or to eliminate undesirable properties in the parent molecule.

Product line extensions They are dosage forms in which the physical form or strength, but not the use or indication, of the product changes. Product line extension is usually performed during clinical phases III, IV, or V.

Production All operations involved in the preparation of an API (active pharmaceutical ingredient), starting from receipt of materials, through processing and packaging, to its completion as a finished API.

Productivity Refers to the amount of production over a given period of time.

Products The compounds that are formed when a reaction goes to completion.

Proembryo Refers to a stage in the early development of the sporophyte between the zygote and the embryo proper, multicellular and globular, but before the differentiation of any tissue systems.

Prokaryote A unicellular organism with less complex structure than a eukaryote, which is characterized by the absence of a nucleus and by having the genetic material in the form of simple filaments of DNA. The sizes of most prokaryotes vary from 0.5 to 3 µm in equivalent radius. Different species have different shapes such as spherical or coccus (staphylococci), cylindrical or bacillus (*E. coli*), or spiral or spirillum (Rhodospirillum).

Prolepsis Refers to the timing of axillary growth, development of an axillary bud only after a period of rest.

Proliferation Refers to an inflorescence which returns to vegetative growth.

Proliferous Bearing supplementary structures like buds or flowers, either in an abnormal manner or in a manner that is normal but from adventitious tissue.

Prominent More or less raised and standing out from the surrounding surface.

Pro-oxidant Any chemical compound, which enhances oxidation.

Propagule A portion of an organism (shoot, leaf, callus, etc.) used for propagation.

Prophage The latent form of a temperate phage, which remains within the lysogen, usually integrated into the host chromosome.

Prophase The first stage of mitosis during that the chromosomes condense, the nuclear envelope disappears, and the centrioles divide and migrate to opposite ends of the cell.

Proportion The expression of the equality of two ratios is a proportion. The product of the extremes is equal to the product of the means for any proportion. Furthermore, the numerator of the one fraction equals the product of its denominator and the other fraction missing term can always be found given the other three terms.

Prophylactic surgery Surgery to remove tissue, which is in danger of becoming cancerous, before cancer has the chance to develop. Surgery to remove the breasts of women at high risk of developing breast cancer is known as prophylactic mastectomy.

Prophylaxis The prevention of, or protective treatment for disease.

Prospective validation Establishing documented evidence, which a system does what it purports to do based on a preplanned protocol.

Prostaglandins A class of fatty acids, which has many of the properties of hormones; synthesized and secreted by many body tissues and have a variety of effects on nearby cells.

Prostheca An extension of a bacterial cell that includes the plasma membrane and cell wall, that is narrower than the mature cell.

Prosthetic groups Refer to organic and/or inorganic components other than amino acids, contained in proteins.

Prostrate Growing on the ground, trailing.

Protease A proteolytic enzyme, which can cleave other proteins into smaller fragments.

Proteasome A large, cylindrical protein complex, which degrades ubiquitin-labeled proteins to

peptides in an ATP-dependent process.

Protectant fungicide Fungicide, which protects a plant from infection by a pathogen.

Protective coverings Any cloth, screen, plastic or other material placed over growing plants to prevent damage by pests or harsh weather.

Protein One of a group of substances constituting the greater part of the nitrogen-containing components of animal and vegetable tissues, very complex constitution, all containing carbon, hydrogen, nitrogen, and oxygen and some containing in addition iron, phosphorus, or sulfur; chemically they are regarded as peptides (polypeptides) or combinations of amino acids and their derivatives. They are colorless, odorless, generally tasteless, and of varying degrees of solubility; they are putrefiable and readily undergo chemical change, hydrolysis, under the influence of ferments and on boiling with dilute acids or alkalis.

Protein engineering The rational design of proteins by constructing specific amino acid sequences through molecular techniques, with the aim of modifying protein characteristics.

Protein sequencer An instrument, which will determine the sequence of amino acids, which make up a particular protein.

Protein splicing Refers to the post-translational process in which part of a precursor polypeptide is removed before the mature polypeptide folds into its final shape. It is carried out by self-splicing proteins that remove inteins and join the remaining exteins.

Proteinoids Polymers of amino acids that are formed spontaneously from inorganic molecules, which have enzyme-like properties and can catalyze chemical reactions.

Proteolysis Protein hydrolysis, the decomposition of protein.

Proteolytic enzyme (protease) Refers to any enzyme, which takes part in the breaking down of proteins. A system of several such enzymes is necessary to breakdown proteins to their constituent amino acids.

Proteome The complete collection of proteins, which an organism produces.

Proteomics A concept more than a defined technology, refers to any protein-based approach, which has the capacity to provide new information about proteins on a genomewide scale. 75% of the predicted proteins in multicellular organisms have no known cellular function.

Prothallus A more or less flattened gametophytic plant body, particularly in bryophytes, ferns and related plants.

Prothorax Refers to the anterior of the three thoracic segments of an insect.

Protists Eucaryotes with unicellular organization, either in the form of solitary cells or colonies of cells lacking true tissues.

Protoalkaloid Refers to an alkaloid that is derived from amino acids, but lacking a heterocyclic ring.

Protocol A prospective plan, which when executed as intended, produces documented evidence that a process or system has been properly qualified.

Protoderm Refers to primary meristem of stem or root, located at the apex, giving rise to the epidermis.

Protogenic (solvent) Capable to act as a proton (hydron) donor strongly or weakly acidic.

Proton Particle found in a nucleus with a positive charge, number of these gives atomic number.

Protophilic (solvent) Capable to act as proton acceptor, strongly or weakly basic.

Protoplasm A semifluid, viscous, translucent mixture of water, proteins, lipids, carbohydrates, and inorganic salts found in all plant and animal cells.

Protoplast A bacterial or fungal cell with its cell wall completely removed, spherical in shape and osmotically sensitive.

Protoplast fusion The joining of cells, which have had their walls weakened or completely removed.

Protostele When a plant's vascular tissue develops in a solid central bundle, it is said to have a protostele.

Prototroph A microorganism, which requires the same nutrients as the majority of naturally occurring members of its species.

Protoxylem Refers to the first formed tissue of the primary xylem differentiating from the procambium, the tracheary cells having spiral or annular thickenings.

Protozoa Nucleated microorganisms, some of which are large enough to be detected with the naked eye, consist of a single cell and/or an aggregation of nondifferentiated cells loosely held together and not forming tissues.

Protuberant Bulging outward provided with pointed, appressed, rigid, hair-like scales or bristles.

Proximal Toward the base, distal.

Pruning Term used for describing the practice of cutting back some or all of the branches of a woody plant. It is done for removing dead or diseased wood for changing plant into a desired shape for promoting vigour of plant in case of fruit trees, for maintaining balance between vegetative growth and fruit formation.

Pruritus Term meaning itching from any cause.

Pseudo (prefix) False, apparent but not genuine.

Pseudoalkaloids Refer to alkaloids derived from terpenes, sterols, aliphatic acids, nicotinic acid, or purines.

Pseudocarp A structure that is made up of the fruit sensu stricto plus another part of the plant, includes everything from rose hips and strawberries to pineapples, figs, and the dispersal units of a dandelion, hardly a term of much value.

Pseudolamina Refers to the extended apical portion of a phyllode.

Pseudoparenchyma Tissue resembling parenchyma with large, thin walled cells, but developmentally filamentous.

Pseudopodium or pseudopod Refers to a nonpermanent cytoplasmic extension of the cell body by which amoebae and amoeboid organisms move and feed.

Psoralen A furanocoumarin.

Psoriasis An autoimmune disorder, which produces red, scaling plaques on the skin that can be associated with mild or severe forms of arthritis.

Psoriatic arthritis Refers to a form of arthritis that is associated with psoriasis.

Psychrophile An organism, which requires temperatures below 20°C (68°F) for growth.

Psychrometer Refers to a hygrometer that uses the difference in readings between two thermometers, one having a wet bulb ventilated to cause evaporation and the other having a dry bulb, as a measure of atmospheric moisture.

Psychrometry For the determination of the properties of gas-vapor mixtures.

Pteridophyte A major division of the plant kingdom, which have clear alternation of generations with a dominant vascular sporophyte initially dependent upon the gametophyte which is very reduced.

Pteridosperm Refers to an extinct group of seed plants which bore fern-like leaves.

Pterocarpans Isoflavonoids, which are derived from isoflavones via oxygenation of the 2'-position.

Ptyxis Pattern of folding and rolling of an individual leaf during early development.

Puberulous Covered with minute, soft, erect hairs.

Pubescent A general term for hairiness, covered with soft hair or down.

Pulverulent Appearing as though dusted over with powder.

Punctate Dotted, with depressed dots scattered over the surface.

Pungent Ending in a stiff, sharp point; with an acrid taste or smell.

Pupa Refers to the non-feeding, inactive stage between larva and adult in insects with complete metamorphosis.

Pupate To molt from the larval stage to the pupa.

Pure culture A culture that contains only one species of microorganism.

Purgative A herb or substance that produces a vigorous and rapid evacuation of the bowels. May also refer to discharges other than from the bowels.

Purified water, USP Water rendered suitable for pharmaceutical purposes by various processes like distillation, ion-exchange treatment (deionization or demineralization), or reverse osmosis.

Purine A nitrogen-containing, double-ring, basic compound, which occurs in nucleic acids, purines in DNA and RNA are adenine and guanine.

Pustule A tiny pus-filled bump on the skin, many pustules can develop on the skin at once.

Putrefaction The microbial decomposition of organic matter, particularly the anaerobic breakdown of proteins, with the production of foul-smelling compounds such as hydrogen sulfide and amines.

Pyoderma gangrenosum Chronic ulcers in the skin often resulting from inflammation diseases inside the body such as inflammatory bowel disease.

Pyrenoid The differentiated region of the chloroplast, which is a center of starch formation in green algae and stoneworts.

Pyridine alkaloids Term used for a group of alkaloids whose structure is based on pyridine nucleus (a 6-membered ring of five carbon and one nitrogen atom and three double bonds).

Pyridine Refers to a toxic, colorless, liquid, aromatic hydrocarbon comprising a substituted benzene ring; pyridine alkaloids are true alkaloids with the parent base being pyridine or lysine.

Pyriform Pear-shaped.

Pyrimidine A nitrogen-containing, single ring, basic compound, which occurs in nucleic acids, the pyrimidines in DNA are cytosine and thymine, in RNA, cytosine, and uracil.

Pyrogen A foreign substance, which produces a fever response in humans and animals, hence the name pyrogen (heat producing). Chemically refers to the lipopolysaccharide outer layer of gram-negative bacteria. Bacterial pyrogens were at one time believed to be toxic substances released when bacterial cells disintegrate and are therefore still referred to as endotoxins.

Pyrolysis Thermolysis, usually associated with exposure to a high temperature.

Pyrrolidine Tetramethylene imine, pyrrolidine alkaloids have a five-membered nitrogen-containing ring.

Pyrrolizidine Refers to a group of alkaloids, based loosely on tropane, via ornithine, containing two fused 5-membered rings with a nitrogen at one of the common positions.

Pyrophoric A chemical, which will spontaneously ignite in air at or below a temperature of 130°F (54.5°C).

Q

QA (quality assurance) The sum total of the organized arrangements made to ensure that all active pharmaceutical ingredients are of the quality required for their intended use and that quality systems are maintained.

QC (quality control) The process involved in testing to ensure if the specifications are met, which the industry measures actual quality performance, compares it with standards, and acts on the difference.

Q fever An acute zoonotic disease caused by the rickettsia *Coxiella burnetii*.

Quality assurance (QA) group The group who interprets the GMP regulations and guidelines.

Quality control (QC) group The group who enforces the GMP regulations.

Quality unit(s) An organizational unit independent of production, which fulfills both quality assurance and quality control responsibilities. This may be in the form of separate QA and QC units, a single individual (or group), depending upon the size and structure of the organization.

Quarantine The grade of materials which is isolated either physically or by other effective means.

Quantitative structure-activity relationships It is a mathematical relationships concerning chemical structure and pharmacological activity in a quantitative manner for a series of compounds.

Quantum Something that comes in separate units.

Quantum numbers It refers to a set of numbers used to illustrate an electron's position.

Quassinoids Refers to a subclass of triterpenoids (nortriterpenoid) having 19-20 carbon atoms.

Quaternary structure The level of structural organization in oligomeric proteins, (i.e. those composed of more than one subunit), which is represented by the number and arrangement of the subunits and the interactions between them.

Quercetin It is a universal flavonol.

Quincuncial The aestivation in a flower such as to facilitate two sepals have one edge outside the adjacent sepal and the other inside, one sepal has both edges inside, and two sepals have both edges outside.

Quinines These are aromatic compounds that have two atoms of hydrogen that are replaced by two atoms of oxygen, generally yellow, red, or orange in colour.

Quinolizidines Alkaloids having two fused 6-membered rings that share nitrogen and are derived from lysine.

Quorum sensing The process in which their own population density is monitored by sensing the levels of signal molecules that are released by the microorganisms. As the signal molecules reach a threshold concentration, the population density attains a critical level or quorum, and quorum-dependent genes are expressed.

R

Rabies An acute infectious disease of the central nervous system, which affects all warm-blooded animals (including humans). It is caused by an ssRNA virus belonging to the genus Lyssavirus in the family Rhabdoviridae.

Race A subdivision of a species, which is capable of interbreeding with other members of the species.

Racemate An equimolar mixture of a pair of enantiomers. It does not exhibit optical activity.

Raceme Inflorescence having a common axis and stalked flowers in acropetel succession.

Racemic Refers to a an equimolar mixture of a pair of enantiomers without any optical activity.

Racemisation The racemate formed from a chiral starting material having an excess enantiomer.

Racemose The inflorescence with no terminal flowers, and the branching is monopodial, as racemes, or spikes as the growing points continue to add to the inflorescence.

Rachis The central prolongation of the stalk called peduncle, or the axis through an inflorescence leaf stalk or through a compound leaf.

Racking The process involved in removing the sediments from wine bottles.

Radappertization The exercise of employing gamma rays from a cobalt source for control of microorganisms in foods.

Radially Arranged like rays emerging equivalently around a central axis.

Radiant energy Energy that is transmitted away from its source.

Radiation Energy in the form of photons.

Radiation sterilization The process of sterilization by means of gamma radiation like cobalt-60, or cesium 137, emitted from radioactive materials.

Radical Positively (radical cation) or negatively (radical anion) molecular entity possessing one or more unpaired electrons, formerly often called "free radical".

Radical centre(s) The atom in a polyatomic radical having an unpaired electron that is basically localized.

Radical ion The radical that carries an electric charge, it could be either positively charged (radical cation) or negatively charged (radical anion).

Radioimmunoassay The process employed to determine the concentration of a substance in the samples, where a purified radioisotope-labeled antigen or antibody is made to compete for antibody or antigen with unlabeled standard and samples.

Radioactive material Any material that can instinctively emits ionizing radiation.

Radioactive decay The spontaneous decay of an atom by emission of alpha and beta decay particle from its nucleus to an atom of a different element.

Radioisotope Term refers radioactive isotope, like carbon-14. Radioisotope nuclei are unstable and suddenly breakdown and emit one of a number of types of radiation.

Ratio The relative magnitude of two like quantities is a ratio, which is expressed as a fraction. Certain basic principles apply to the ratio, as they do to all fractions.

Ratio strength Solid or liquid formulations that contain low concentrations of active ingredients will often have concentration expressed in ratio strength. Ratio strength, as the name implies, is the expression of concentration by means of ratio.

Raw material A general term used to represent the starting materials, reagents, intermediates, process aids, and solvents proposed for use in the construction of intermediates or active pharmaceutical ingredients (API).

Reactants Substances that are present in the beginning of a chemical reaction.

Reaction wood Wood formed at the position where branch joins the stem, they often have a characteristic anatomy.

Reactive oxygen species Molecules like superoxide radical that can cause a damage or other highly reactive forms of oxygen (like singlet oxygen) that can harm biomolecules and facilitate in disease states.

Reactivity index Any numerical index derived from quantum mechanical model calculations

that authorize the prediction of relative reactivities of different molecular sites.

Reagent Any substance used for the purpose of detecting or measuring a component, or for preparing a product, because of its chemical or biological activity.

Reagin Antibody that mediates immediate hypersensitivity reactions. IgE is the major reagin that occurs in humans.

Receptacle Somewhat prolonged apex of a floral axis with the floral parts.

Receptor A chemical group available on the cell surface or interior to accept the stimuli from a specific chemical group, molecule, or virus.

Receptor mapping The technique used to express the geometric and electronic features of a binding site when inadequate structural data for receptor or enzyme are available.

Recessive allele A gene, which is expressed only when its counterpart allele on the matching chromosome is also recessive (not dominant).

Recombinant Refers to the recombining of generic material from one species into alternate sequences.

Recombinant DNA technology The techniques involved the identification and isolation of a specific gene, the insertion of the gene into a vector for instance a plasmid to form a recombinant molecule, and the production of large quantities of the gene and its products.

Recombinant-vector vaccine The category of vaccine that is created by putting together of one or more of a pathogen's genes into attenuated viruses or bacteria. The attenuated virus or bacterium serves as a vector, replicating within the vertebrate host and expressing the gene(s) of the pathogen. The pathogen's antigens induce an immune response.

Recombinant clone Clone containing recombinant DNA molecules.

Recombinant DNA (RDNA) The hybrid DNA created by unification of pieces of DNA from different sources.

Recovery The process intended to make any material suitable for further use.

Recurved Any thing that is curved or curled downwards or backwards.

Redfield ratio The carbon-nitrogen-phosphorus ratio of aquatic microorganisms and the ratio plays an prime role as it predicts the limiting factors for microbial growth.

Red algae Common name for the algae coming under the division Rhodophyta.

Red tides Red tides occur often in coastal areas and often are associated with population blooms of dinoflagellates. Dinoflagellate pigments are the one responsible for the red color of the water. Under these conditions, the dinoflagellates often produce saxitoxin, which can lead to paralytic shellfish poisoning.

Redox potential Any oxidation-reduction (redox) reaction can be divided into two half reactions: one in which a chemical species undergoes oxidation and one in which another chemical species undergoes reduction. The redox potential is the reduction/oxidation potential of a compound measured under standard conditions against a standard reference half-cell.

Reducing agent or reductant The electron donor in an oxidation-reduction reaction.

Reduction reaction A reaction in which a substance gains at least one electron.

Reference drug product The reference drug product is usually the currently marketed, brand name product with a full new drug application (NDA) approved by the FDA.

Reference standard An authentic material with high purity.

Reflex An involuntary response to stimulate the body.

Reflexology The treatment employed in the basis of the idea that specific points on the feet and hands correspond with organs and tissues throughout the body. With fingers and thumbs, the practitioner applies pressure to these points to treat a wide range of stress-related illnesses and ailments.

Refrigerant The herb or material that facilitates a cooling feeling to the mucous membranes, and reduces abnormal body heat and fever. Externally, it cools by evaporation or fluids used for heat transfer in a refrigerating system; the refrigerant absorbs heat and transfers it at a higher temperature and higher pressure, usually with a change of state.

Refraction The deflection of a light ray from a straight path when it get ahead from one medium to another.

Refractive index The ratio of the velocity of light in the first of two media to that in the second as it passes from the first to the second.

Regimen Exactingly regulated course of medication intended to achieve best possible results.

Region of division Refers to the area of cell division in the tip of a plant root.

Region of elongation The area in the tip of a plant root where cells grow by elongating, thus increasing the length of the root.

Region of maturation Refers to the area where primary tissues and root hairs develop in the tip of a plant root.

Regulatory affairs Drug companies must show that their products consistently meet standards set by government agencies. Regulatory affairs departments document those activities, submit proposals, and follow those proposals through completion or approval.

Regulatory sequence A DNA base sequence that controls gene expression.

Reiteration Refers to plant architecture, when the characteristic construction of the individual is repeated by branch systems that develop on a plant after damage, or sometimes as the result of natural causes.

Relapse An exacerbation or period of time when symptoms worsen. These periods may come and go without warning and may last a few days or weeks at a time.

Relative bioavailability Relative bioavailability is the systemic availability of the drug from a dosage form as compared to a reference standard given by the same route of administration. Relative bioavailability is calculated as the ratio of the AUC for the reference dosage form given in the same dose.

Relative humidity (% RH) The ratio (measured in percent) of actual water vapor pressure in air to the pressure of saturated water vapor in air at the same temperature and pressure.

Relaxant A herb or substance that relaxes, eases, and relieves tension and strain.

Remission A period of time when symptoms lessen.

Remote Separated from one another; separated by intervals or spaces greater than the ordinary.

Renal clearance Renal clearance is the volume of drug contained in the plasma that is removed by the kidney per unit time. Units for renal clearance are expressed in volume per time, (e.g. millimeters per minute or litre per hour).

Reniform Having the form or shape of a kidney.

Renin An enzyme, which is secreted by the kidneys that converts angiotensinogen into angiotensin II.

Repeat-action tablets Repeat-action tablets are layered or compression-coated tablets in which the outer layer or shell rapidly disintegrates in the stomach. The components of the inner layer or inner tablet are insoluble in gastric media, but soluble in intestinal media.

Replication The process in which an exact copy of parental DNA or RNA is made with the parental molecule serving as a template.

Repressor protein A protein coded for by a regulator gene that can bind to the operator and inhibit transcription; it may be active by itself or only when the corepressor is bound to it.

Reproductive system One of eleven major body organ systems in animals; is responsible for reproduction and thus the survival of the species.

Resin These are natural organic substances formed as plant secretions either solid or semi-solid in appearance, flammable, soluble in organic solvents. The resins are complex chemical mixtures of acrid resins, resin alcohols, resinol, tannols, esters, and resenes.

Resina The resin that is obtained from a plant or by distillation of the balsamum.

Resistant Any able to tolerate conditions.

Respiration The process by which nutrients are oxidized externally to provide energy required for cellular activity.

Respiratory burst An activated phagocytic cell increases its oxygen consumption to support the increased metabolic activity of phagocytosis, which leads to respiratory burst. It generates highly toxic oxygen products such as singlet oxygen, superoxide radical, hydrogen peroxide, hydroxyl radical, and hypochlorite.

Respiratory system One among the eleven major system in animals that akesmoves oxygen from the external environment into the internal environment and expels out carbon dioxide from the body.

Restriction endonuclease Restriction endonuclease is an enzyme that cleaves DNA at sequence-specific sites.

Reticulate Interlocked, similar to a network.

Retinol Also called vitamin A.

Retinopathy An abnormality of or damage to the retina layer of the eye.

Retinoblastoma An eye cancer which typically appears in childhood due to the reason that a pair of tumor-suppressor genes is missing from birth.

Retrorse When the hairs are turned toward the base.

Retrospective validation Establishing documented evidence that a system does what it claims to do based on review and analysis of historic information.

Retroviruses A group of viruses with RNA genomes, which carry the enzyme reverse transcriptase and form a DNA copy of their genome during their reproductive cycle.

Retuse Having a shallow, rounded notch at the apex.

Reverse osmosis (RO) The reversal of osmosis to purify water. The flow of water can be reversed with an opposing pressure that exceeds osmotic pressure.

Reverse transcriptase An RNA-dependent DNA polymerase that uses a viral RNA genome as a template to form a DNA copy; this is a reverse of the normal flow of genetic information, which proceeds from DNA to RNA.

Reye's syndrome An acute, fatal disease occurring in children with severe edema in brain, increased intracranial pressure, vomiting, hypoglycemia, and liver dysfunction.

Rheumatic fever It is an autoimmune disease associated with hemolytic streptococci in the body, with symptoms of inflammatory lesions involving the heart valves, joints, subcutaneous tissues, and central nervous system. The disease is called as rheumatic fever because both fever and pain in the joints as similar to that of rheumatism occurs.

Rheumatic disease A disease having pain or inflammation in the musculoskeletal system like bones, joints, muscles, tendons, and ligaments.

Rheumatic skin disease Skin problems occurring due to rheumatic disease.

Rheumatoid arthritis A rigorous type of autoimmune arthritis, , if not properly treated can destroy the joints.

Rhizoid The cellular outgrowth of a plant that usually assist in affixing to the surface and increasing surface area to gain water or nutrients; found in mosses, liverworts, and hornworts.

Rhizoma Relates to rhizome or horizontal stem, usually consisting of roots on its underside.

Rhizomatous tuber Otherwise called corm.

Rhizome The horizontal root-like stem having leaves and shoots produced from its upper surface and roots from its lower surface.

Rhizosphere The segment surrounding the plant root with increased microbial population and its activities.

Rhytidome Cork cambium and the tissues it isolates, since such cambia are often formed successively deeper in the stem, there may be pockets of cortical or phloem tissue in the cork.

Ribonucleic acid A polynucleotide consisting of ribonucleotides united by phosphodiester bridges.

Ribosomal RNA The RNA present in ribosomes that are directly involved in the mechanism of protein synthesis. Ribosomes contain numerous single-stranded rRNA that take part in the structure of ribosome.

Ribosome Refers to the organelle where protein synthesis occurs and the message encoded in mRNA is translated here.

Ribonucleic acids (RNA) Linear polymer molecules, which are composed of a chain of ribose units linked between positions 3 and 5 by phosphodiester groups (the molecules that translate the genetic code from DNA to produce proteins). The three important types of RNAs in the cell are messenger RNA (mRNA), transfer RNA (tRNA) and ribosomal RNA (rRNA).

Rickettsias Gram-negative microorganisms that are smaller than other bacteria and are carried by arthropod vectors and can infect both human and other mammal. They require living cells for growth.

RNA polymerase The enzyme that catalyzes the synthesis of mRNA through the path of a DNA template.

Root The non-green part of a plant, functioning as to grip the plant in position, draws water and nutrients from the soil, stores food.

Root cap The collection of cells that envelops the apical meristem of the root.

Root hair The projection from an epidermal cell of the root.

Root pressure The pressure developed within the roots due to the liquid secreation from the root stump, when the shoot is cut off.

Root tip The apical portion of the root along with the apical meristem and root cap.

Root tuber Swollen food or storing roots.

Rootlet The small root or small branch of a root.

Rootstock The underground stem or rhizome; that grows into the root system.

Rosette Series of whorls of leaves like structure formed at the bottom of the stem.

Rotation The practice of cultivating an alternating crop in the same land.

Rotenoids Flavonoids obtained by the addition of an extra carbon atom from S-adenosyl methionine and in prenyl group into the isoflavone structure.

Routes of administration The way through which a drug is administered into the body.

Rubber One of the constituent of latex with cis 1,4-polyisoprene.

Rubefacient The agent ment to relieve internal pain by applying tropically due to local irritation and redness.

Rubiaceous Also called paracytic type of stomata.

Rudimentary That which is not developed completely and is not functional.

Rue leaf The leaf produced after the cotyledons.

Rugose Virus infections resulting in rough look of leaves, and also the veins become sunken and interveinal tissue are raised.

Ruminant The hoofed mammals like cattle or deer that chew the cud.

Ruminate Term pertaining to endosperm, inpushings of the seed coat, which more or less give the appearance of the villi of the rumen or intestine to the cut surface of the seed.

Runner The slender, prostrate ground stem which produces roots and erect shoots at their nodes.

Ruspolinone Refers to pyrrolidine alkaloid.

Russeting Thickening of the periderm that occurs after vine senescence on tubers of russet cultivars.

S

S phase Refers to the period of interphase when new DNA is synthesized as a part of replication of the chromatin.

Saccate In the form of a sac or pouch.

Saccharose Sucrose.

Safranin A base, obtained from aniline; aniline pink; used as a stain in histology.

Sagittate In the form of its head like an arrow and the basal lobes pointing down.

Salicylic acid Orthohydroxybenzoic acid as salicylate salts are obtained from the bark of the white willow and wintergreen leaves.

Salmonellosis An infection caused by some species of the genus Salmonella, through food contaminated with salmonellae or their products. It is also called *Salmonella gastroenteritis* or *Salmonella* food poisoning.

Salt A compound formed by the interaction of an acid and a base, the hydrogen atoms of the acid being replaced by another positive ion derived from the base.

Salve Herbal formulation prepared by mixing in oil and thickened with bees wax, used for applying to the skin.

Sandy crystal Refers to a microcrystalline form of calcium oxalate, or some other crystalline inclusion that forms a granular mass.

Sanitation The measures taken or the activity done to reduce the spread of pathogen inoculum, e.g. removal and destruction of infected plant parts.

Sanitization Reducing the microbial population on an inanimate object to levels judged safe by public health standards.

Sap The aqueous liquid found in the xylem and phloem vessels containing mineral salts, sugars and other organic substances.

Saponification Alkaline hydrolysis of triacyl glycerols to yield fatty acids as soaps.

Saponin The surfactant glycosides found in plants, which can produce soapy lather.

Saprophyte The organisms that feed on nonliving organic nutrients in dissolved form and grows on decomposing organic matter.

Saprozoic nutrition The nutrition that includes organic nutrients are in dissolved form, e.g. animals or animal-like organisms.

Sapwood The outer and nonfunctional region of the wood in a trunk or large root.

Sarcotesta The fleshy layer of the testa (mesotesta), outside the sclerotesta, when the sclerotesta is present.

Sarmentose The plant with thin runners.

Saturated air When there is a state of mutual equilibrium between the moist air and the liquid or solid phases of water. Saturated air holds as much water vapor as it can for a given temperature and pressure.

Saturated fat A fat having single covalent bonds between the carbons of its fatty acids.

Saturated fatty acids Fatty acids containing fully saturated alkyl chains.

Saturated solutions Saturated solutions are solutions which, at a given temperature and pressure, contain the maximum amount of solute that can be accommodated by the solvent.

Saturation humidity The air is saturated when the partial pressure of water vapor in the air at a given temperature equals the vapor pressure of water at the same temperature.

Saxicolous That which can living on a rock.

Saxitoxin The neurotoxins produced by dinoflagellate *Gonyaulax*.

Scabrate The term used to express the pollen surface, ornamented with elements less than 1μm in all directions.

Scabrid Somewhat rough.

Scabrous Rough to the touch.

Scalariform With a ladder-like pattern in a vessel.

Scale The plate-like organic structure seen on the surface of some cells.

Scale-up To take a biopharmaceutical manufacturing process from the laboratory scale to a scale at which it is commercially feasible.

Scale leaf The reduced, frequently dry, non-photosynthetic and protective leaf, e.g. surrounding a dormant bud, a budscale.

Scanning electron microscope (SEM) The electron microscope can scans a beam of electrons over the surface of a specimen and produce an image from the electrons that are emitted by the surface.

Scarious Any object that is tough, thin, dry, and semitransparent.

Scarlet fever A communicable disease (through respiratory droplets) caused by the infection of strain of *Streptococcus pyogenes* that carries a lysogenic phage with the gene for erythrogenic (rash-inducing) toxin resulting in shedding of the skin.

Scarring Permanent disfigurement of tissues due to some type of injury.

Scavenger A substance that reacts with (or otherwise removes) a trace component or traps a reactive reaction intermediate (as in the scavenging of radicals or free electrons).

Schizocarp The dry fruit, that splits at maturity into two or more parts with one seeded carpels which remain closed.

Schizogenous The cavity present in plants, formed by the partition of cells through their middle lamellae.

Schizogony The process of multiple asexual fission.

Sclereid Sclerenchyma consist of sclerides as the dead cells are highly lignified wall.

Sclerenchyma Highly lignified tissue with uniformly thick walled, dead cells in the stem whose principal function is mechanical. They are clustered into fibers.

Scleromorphic The hardness or toughness of a leaves due to dry climate or nutrient poor conditions.

Sclerosis Hardening of tissue.

Sclerotesta The sclerenchyma-tous layer of the testa, generally mesotestal in origin and inside the sarcotesta.

Sclerotium The hard compact mass of mycelium that acts as a dormant stage in some fungi.

Scopoletin The coumarin.

Scurvy The deficiency disease caused by vitamin C. It is charac-terized by rotting gums, loosened teeth, and bleeding skin and mucous membranes.

Second law of thermodynamics (entropy) The energy available after a chemical reaction is less than that at the beginning of a reaction; energy conversions are not 100% efficient.

Secondary growth Growth that occurs wood and bark in seed plants, which results after elongation and maturation of the primary tissues is completed.

Secondary infection Those infec-tions that are caused due to the infection by microorganisms that enter the host through an injury previously produced by another pathogen.

Secondary meristem It is also called lateral meristem.

Secondary metabolites The meta-bolism during which some pro-ducts are formed that are not essential for normal growth, development and reproduction, but generally are important in there ecological function.

Secondary phloem Phloem that is produced by the vascular cambium in a woody plant stem or root.

Secondary roots The arrangement of very thin roots that come from the primary roots of a strawberry plant and take water and nutri-ents from the soil; white roots.

Secondary stems Stems pro-duced from stolons that come out from the soil.

Secondary thickening Diameter of the stem is increase due to the of the activity of the lateral meristems.

Secondary tissue The distin-guished products of lateral meristems.

Secondary xylem Xylem that is produced by the vascular cam-bium in a woody plant stem or root.

Secretory It refers to glandular.

Sedative Any herb or substance that has the ability of reducing the nervous tension.

Sediment Loose aggregate of solids that are derived from pre-existing rocks, or solids precipi-tated from solution by inorganic chemical processes.

Sedimentary rock Refers to any rock composed of sediment, i.e. solid particles and dissolved min-erals, e.g. rocks, which form from sand or mud in riverbeds or on the sea bottom.

Seed The portion of a flowering plant having the embryo and can be germinate if sown.

Seed coat The outer cover of a seed.

Seed cotton Lint that is attached to seeds even after harvesting.

Seed leaf It refers to cotyledon.

Seedling The newly formed plant after the germination of the seed.

Segmented genome The genome of virus that is separated into numerous fragments, each coding for the synthesis of a single poly-peptide. These types of segmented genomes are extremely common among the RNA viruses.

Selective breeding Refers to the selection of individuals with desirable traits for use in breeding.

Selective media Culture media that support the development of a particular microorganism with the inhibition in growth of undesired microorganisms.

Selective pesticide Those pesticides that are poisonous mainly to the target pest and its related species with no harmful effect to other organisms, including natural enemies.

Selenium The mineral with the ability to alter the course of cancer by serving some enzymes protect cells against damage.

Self-pollination The process of pollination by pollen of a flower in same plant.

Semipermeable Membranes, which do not have measurable pores but through which smaller molecules can pass.

Senecionine It refers to pyrrolizidine alkaloid.

Senescence The stage of growth in a plant or plant part, which refers from maturity to death and is characterized by an accumulation of metabolic products, an increased respiratory rate, and a loss in dry weight.

Sensory neuropathy Numbness and tingling primarily sensed in the arms, legs, hands, and feet due to the damage of nerves that provide sensation to these parts of the body.

Sepal One among the outmost part in the structures of flower having other flower parts enclosed in it as the bud.

Sepaloid Having the appearance as like a sepal, e.g. of bracts, when green and arranged in a ring beneath a flower.

Sepsis Systemic response to infection occurring due to the presence of pathogens or their toxins in blood and other tissues.

Septate That which is divided by a septum or septa.

Septic shock Sepsis that is associated with severe hypotension in spite of adequate fluid resuscitation, along with the presence of perfusion abnormalities, which may include, lactic acidosis, oliguria, or an acute alteration in mental status. Gram-positive bacteria, fungi, and endotoxin-containing gram-negative bacteria can initiate the pathogenic flow of sepsis leading to septic shock.

Septum The separation or cross-wall presents between two cells in a bacterium.

Sequential sampling The process of sampling method where prior fixation on the number of samples is not done.

Serology The branch of immunology that deals with *in vitro* reactions connecting to one or more serum constituents, e.g. antibodies and complement.

Serotonin The neurotransmitter (empirical formula $C_{10}H_{12}N_2O$) believed to be active in regulating body temperature and sleep pattern.

Serrate Refers to leaves margins, notched on edge like a saw or having sharp notches along the edge pointing toward the apex.

Serum The clear, liquid fraction remaining after coagulation of plasma, deficient of blood cells and fibrinogen. It is the noncellular liquid faction of blood.

Serum resistance The type of resistance, which occurs with bacteria such as *Neisseria gonorrhoeae* because the pathogen interferes with membrane attack complex formation during the complement cascade.

Sesamin It refers to lignan.

Sesquiterpene lactones Refers to lactones, subclass of C15 terpenoids (sesquiterpenoids, sesquiterpenes), bitter tasting and toxic, which are derived via the mevalonate pathway from three C5 isopentenyl pyrophosphate units.

Sessile The leaf without a stalk, pedicel, or peduncle.

Seta Stiff hair, projection or bristle

Sex chromosomes Chromosomes, which determine the sex of an organism. In humans, females have two X chromosomes, and males have one X and one Y chromosome.

Sex pilus A thin protein attachment necessary for bacterial mating or conjugation. The cell having sex pili represents DNA to recipient cells.

Sexual reproduction A reproduction system in which two haploid sex cells fuse to produce a diploid zygote.

Sheath Tubelike structure that is hallow and is surrounding a chain of cells and present in several genera of bacteria.

Shells The 4 types of electron shells: s, p, d and f shells, where the electrons generally stay.

Shiatsu The type of acupressure, used in Japan for the treatment of stress, circulatory problems, headaches, asthma, diarrhea, bronchitis, depression. It has been followed in Japan for over 1,000 years.

Shielding As per NMR spectroscopy, shielding is the effect of the electron shells of the observed and the neighbouring nuclei on the external magnetic field. The external field induces circulations in the electron cloud. The resulting magnetic moment is oriented in the opposite direction to the external field, so that the local field at the central nucleus is weakened, although it may be strengthened at other nuclei (deshielding).

Shigellosis The bacillary dysentery caused by a species belonging to the genus Shigella.

Shikimic acid The aromatic carboxylic acid that acts as a precursor in the biosynthesis of alkaloids and flavonoids.

Shingles The reactivated type of chickenpox caused by the *varicella-zoster* virus.

Shoot The portion of a plant above the soil consisting of leaves, flowers, fruits, etc.

Short-day plant The group of plant having a need of less than 12 hours of daylight for flowering.

Shrub The woody plants with high less than five metres, without a separate main axis, or the branches arising on the main axis more or less from the base.

SI unit Refers Systeme International d'Unites, a international system that established a uniform set of measurement units.

Sialogogue The herb or drug that has the ability to stimulate secretion of saliva.

Side dressing Fertilizer or other supplementary put to the soil surrounding a growing crop.

Side effect The problems that arises due to the treatment of another disease.

Sieve cell These are a conducting cell in phloem tissue of gymnosperms.

Sieve element The cell in phloem tissue concerned with the longitudinal conduction of food materials.

Sieve plate The particular area on the wall of a sieve tube having large pores than that are found anywhere else on the wall.

Sigma bonds A covalent bond with the electrons located in between the nuclei.

Sigma factor The protein that facilitate the RNA polymerase core enzyme to recognize the promoter at the beginning of a gene.

Silage Refers to the fermented plant material with increased palatability and nutritional value for animals that can be stored for extended period.

Silent mutation The mutation without any change in the proteins or phenotype of an organism's, irrespective of the fact that the DNA base sequence has been changed.

Siliceous Having silica (SiO_2).

Silicoflagellate Chrysophycean organism bearing silicious skeleton.

Simillimum The most similar remedy corresponding to a case.

Simple fruit Fruit made from either a single carpel or by two or more connate carpels.

Simple leaf The leaf devoid of leaflets.

Sinapine, sinigrine Methyl glucosinolates.

Single bond When an electron pair is shared by two different elements.

Sinuate Containing a wavy margin, like few leaves.

Sister chromatids Chromatids joined by a common centromere and that carries identical genetic information.

Skeletal muscle Muscle that is normally associated with the skeleton and support the movement of the body parts.

Skeletal system The organ system in animals, that supports the body, protects internal organs, allows movement of the body.

Skotophilic Dark loving.

Slaked lime Calcium hydroxide, $Ca(OH)_2$.

Slime The viscous extracellular glycoproteins or glycolipids produced by some bacteria, which allow them to adhere to smooth surfaces such as prosthetic medical devices and catheters. Generally this term often refers to an easily removed, diffuse, unorganized layer of extracellular material that surrounds a bacterial cell.

Slit The stretched out opening from which pollen escapes from an anther.

Slough Refers to wet place of deep mud, a sluggish channel, a swamp, bog, or marsh, especially one that is part of an inlet or backwater.

Sludge A general term for the precipitated solid matter produced during water and sewage treatment; solid particles composed of organic matter and microorganisms that are involved in aerobic sewage treatment (activated sludge).

Small intestine A coiled tube in the abdominal cavity, which is the major site of chemical digestion and absorption of nutrients. It is composed of duodenum, jejunum, and ileum.

Smallpox The disease characterized by skin eruptions and pustules that is caused by the poxvirus.

Smooth muscle Muscles without striations and are found around vessels and in the walls of circulatory system like stomach, intestines, and bladder.

Soda Sodium carbonate, Na_2CO_3.

Soft drug A soft drug is a compound, which is degraded *in vivo* to predictable non-toxic and inactive metabolites, after achieving its therapeutic role.

Soil Tough rocks and minerals combined with air, water and organic matter, which can support plants.

Solarization Refers to the practice of heating soil to levels lethal to pests through application of clear plastic to the soil surface for 4 to 6 weeks during sunny, warm weather.

Solid extract An extract of plant material(s) made by removing the solvent from a liquid extract.

Solitary Borne singly, not grouped.

Solute Refers to any substance dissolved in a solution, e.g. the salt in saltwater.

Solution It is a homogeneous mixture composed of one or more substances, known as solutes, dissolved in another substance, known as a solvent.

Solvation Refers to any stabilizing interaction of a solute and the solvent or a similar interaction with solvent of groups of an insoluble material.

Solvent Refers to liquid in which something is dissolved, e.g. the water in saltwater.

Solvolysis Reaction with a solvent that involves the rupture of one or more bonds in the reacting solute.

Somatic Term used for describing all parts of a plant, apart from the germ mother-cells and gametes.

Somatic apogamy Refers to the development of the sporophyte from the tissues of a gametophyte, without involving the fusion of nuclei. It therefore has the same chromosome number as the gametophyte.

Somatic cell Refers to any cell of the vegetative body of the organism other than reproductive cell, i.e. spore, gamete or their precursors.

Somatic embryo An embryo developing from previously differentiated somatic cells, not from a zygote.

Somatic hybridization Refers to the production of cells tissues or organisms by involving fusion of non-gametic nuclei. Inducing fusion in cells that normally never fuse together and, finds use in plant breeding or genetics.

Somatic nervous system Refers to the portion of the peripheral nervous system consisting of the motor neuron pathways that innervate skeletal muscles.

Sonication Irradiation with (often ultra)sound waves, to increase the rate of a reaction or to prepare vesicles in mixtures of surfactants and water or to extract out phytoconstituents.

SOP (standard operating procedure) The description of necessary activities to respond to normal and abnormal situations in an operating system. SOPs should also describe normal operation, maintenance, and cleaning of the system, and normal operating parameters. Also the SOP may include a troubleshooting checklist, list of personnel to contact, etc.

Soporific A herb or substance that induces sleep.

Sorbitol A hexitol, which is formed by reduction of the carbonyl group of glucose.

Southern blotting technique Refers to the procedure that is used to isolate and identify DNA fragments from a complex mixture. The isolated, denatured fragments are transferred from an agarose electrophoretic gel to a nitrocellulose filter and then identified by hybridization with probes.

Spasticity An abnormal increase in muscle tone that leads to muscle stiffness and rigidity.

Spathe A large leaf-like part or pair of such that encloses a flower cluster.

Spatulate As the shape of some leaves, shaped like a spatula or spoon, gradually widening distally and with a rounded tip.

Speciation The chemical form or compound in which an element occurs in both non-living and living systems, also the quantitative distribution of an element. In biology, it refers to the origination of a new species.

Species This is the level that defines an individual plant. Often, the name will describe some aspect of the plant—the colour of the flowers, size or shape of the leaves, or it may be named after the place where it was found. Together, the genus and species name refer to only one plant, and they are used to identify that particular plant. Also term refers to group of interbreeding individuals, not interbreeding with another such group, being a taxonomic unit including two names in binomial nomenclature, the generic name and specific epithet, similar and related species being grouped into a genus.

Specific catalysis The acceleration of a reaction by a exclusive catalyst, than by a family of related substances.

Specific heat Refers to the amount of heat it takes for a substance to be raised 1°C.

Specification A list of tests, references to analytical procedures, and appropriate acceptance criteria which are numerical limits, ranges, or other criteria for the tests described.

Sperm The male reproductive cell, the male gamete, sperm is mostly a nucleus surrounded by little other cellular material. In plants, the two nuclei of the male gametophyte of angiosperms that are produced from the generative cell.

Spermatophyta It is a major division of the plant kingdom, characterized by reproducing by seed and it is subdivided into the Gymnospermae and Angiospermae.

Spermosphere The region that surrounds a germinating seed where released organic matter stimulates microbial growth.

Spherical Sphere-shaped, a general pollen shape descriptor.

Spheroplast A relatively spherical cell formed by the weakening or partial removal of the rigid cell wall component, (e.g. by antibiotic treatment of gram-negative bacteria), usually osmotically sensitive.

Spicate With the form of a spike.

Spicule Small, slim, pointed portion, typically found on a surface.

Spike Flower cluster that is stretched attached directly to the stalk.

Spin density The unpaired electron density at a position of interest, generally at carbon, in a radical.

Spin trapping It is a technique for detecting short-lived reactive free radicals in biological systems by providing a nitrone or nitrose compound for an addition reaction to occur that produces an electron spin resonance spectroscopy-detectable aminoxyl radical. In spin trapping, the compound trapping the radical is called the spin trap and the addition product of the radical is identified as the spin adduct.

Spinal cord Refers to the thick longitudinal cord of nervous tissue, which extends along the back in on top of the vertebrae. It serves not only as a pathway for nervous impulses to and from the brain but as a center for carrying out and coordinating many reflex actions independently of the brain.

Spine Refers to a stiff, vascularised, sharp pointed structure, formed from a leaf or part of a leaf such as a stipule, leaf tooth, etc.

Spin-spin coupling The interaction involving the spin magnetic moments of diverse electrons or nuclei.

Spiracle The external opening of the system of ducts, or tracheae which functions as respiratory system in insects.

Spirillum Spiral-shaped bacterium that is rigid.

Spirits Spirits, or essences, are alcoholic or hydro-alcoholic solutions of volatile substances that contain 50–90% alcohol.

Spirochete Spiral-shaped bacterium with periplasmic flagella that is flexible.

Spleen It is a secondary lymphoid organ that function to destroy the old erythrocytes and trap the blood-borne antigens and present them to lymphocytes.

Split or interrupted gene Structural gene with DNA sequences that code for the final RNA product separated by regions coding for RNA absent from the mature RNA.

Spongiform encephalopathies The diseases resulting in the degenerative central nervous system in brain, giving it a soft appearance due to prions.

Spongy Mesophyll of leaf, where the cells are little elongated and packed with large intercellular spaces.

Spontaneous generation The hypothesis that living organisms can arise from nonliving matter.

Spontaneous reaction The reaction that will continue even without any exterior energy.

Sporadic disease A disease that takes place rarely but at random intervals in a population.

Sporangiospore The spore that are born within a sporangium.

Sporangium A chamber where the spores are produced during meiosis.

Spore The cell that does not act as a gamete but still function in reproduction.

Sporocyte The cell that produces spores by undergoing meiosis.

Sporogenous The process of generation of spore.

Sporophyll The leaf with the ability of bearing sporangia is called a sporophyll.

Sporophyte These are plants that bears spores formed by meiosis.

Sporotrichosis A subcutaneous fungal infection caused by the dimorphic fungus, *Sporothrix schenckii*.

Sporulation The process of formation of spore.

Spread plate The petri dish containing a solid culture medium having isolated microbial colonies growing on its surface, by spreading a dilute microbial suspension evenly over the agar surface.

Spring wood Refers to as early wood.

Sprout New stem produced from the eye of a potato tuber.

Spur Tube-like structure produced by an extension of one or more petals or sepals; also refers to a very short branch with closely spaced leaves.

Sputum The mucous secretion expelled through the mouth from the lungs, bronchi, and trachea.

Stalk Nonliving bacterial appendage produced by the cell and extending from it.

Stability Generally, stability refers to the physico-chemical condition of a parenteral, biological, or shelf-life of labile drugs.

Stamens The male reproductive structures of a flower, generally consist of slender, thread-like filaments topped by anthers.

Standard free energy change The free energy change of a reaction at 1 atmosphere pressure when all reactants and products are present in their standard states; usually the temperature is 25°C.

Standard reduction potential A measure of the tendency of a reductant to lose electrons in an oxidation-reduction (redox) reaction. The more negative the reduction potential of a compound, the better electron donor it is.

Stability constant The equilibrium constant that states the propensity of a species to form from its component parts. The greater the stability constant, the more stable is the species.

Stable The term describing the state of equilibrium matching to a local minimum of the appropriate thermodynamic potential for the specified constraints on the system.

Staggered conformation The conformation of groups attached to two adjacent atoms is said to be staggered if the *torsion angles* are such that the groups are as far away as possible from an eclipsed arrangement.

Stalk The stem of a plant, that supports the leaves, flowers, and fruit.

Stamen The male reproductive organs in flowers, with the filament, and the anther, filled with pollen, located within the petals.

Staminate Flowers consisting of stamens but not pistils.

Staminate flower Male flower.

Standardisation Adjusting the drug preparation to a defined content of a constituent or a group of substances with known therapeutic activity respectively by adding excipients or by mixing herbal drug preparations. In some member states, the expression "standardisation" is used on a national level to describe all measures which are taken during the manufacturing process and quality control leading to a reproducible quality.

Standardize Evaluation of a concentrated botanical extract to find the amount of the determined levels of 'marker' guaranteed to be present in every batch.

Starch sheath The outer layer of cells of a two-layered bundle sheath containing starch that surrounds the vascular bundle.

Starch The coiled chain polysaccharide prepared from alpha glucose units.

Starter culture The inoculum consisting of cautiously chosen microorganisms, used for the purpose of starting a commercial fermentation.

Stationary phase Refers to the phase of microbial growth in a batch culture when population growth ceases and the growth curve levels off.

Statistics The mathematics involved in the collection, organization, and interpretation of numerical data.

Staurocytic Stomata having three to five subsidiary cells and each oblique to the long axis of the guard cells.

Steady state If during the course of a chemical reaction, the concentration of an intermediate remains constant, than the intermediate is said to be in a steady state.

Steady-state volume of distribution The steady-state volume of distribution is the amount of drug in the body at steady state the average steady-state drug concentration.

Steam distilling The process employed to extract out the volatile principles from the plant. Plant material is either boiled in water or steam is passed through it so that the volatiles are carried off in the steam and recovered in a condenser.

Stele The central cylinder consisting of vascular tissue with xylem, phloem and pericycle and in a few cases pith and medullary rays, inside the cortex of the roots and stems of vascular plants.

Stellate Star-like branch in a way as to radiate from a central point.

Stem The major axis of a plant above the soil surface, having leaves with characteristic arrangement of the vascular tissue.

Stem-nodulating rhizobia Rhizobia which produce nitrogen-fixing structures above the soil surface on plant stems.

Stem tuber Swollen structures produced by stolons and runners that remain dormant during adverse conditions and later grow into new plants when the conditions become favorable for growth.

Steno Refers to narrow.

Stereochemical Viewing of three-dimensional molecule as such or in a projection.

Stereoconvergence The predominant formation of the same stereoisomer or stereoisomer mixture of a reaction product when two different stereoisomers of the reactant are used in the same reaction. When that product involved in the reaction is one enantiomer the result has been called enantioconvergence.

Stereoisomer Two molecules are 'stereoisomers' of each other when they have the exact numbers and kinds of atoms that are bonded to each other in the same order but do differ in the bonds orientation in space.

Stereoisomeric Isomerism that occurs due to difference in the spatial arrangement of atoms without any variation in bond multiplicity between the isomers.

Stereomutation The change of configuration at a stereogenic *unit* brought due to physical or chemical means.

Stereoselective synthesis Chemical reaction in which one or more new elements of chirality are formed in a substrate molecule and which produces enantiomeric or diastereoisomeric in unequal amounts.

Stereospecificity A reaction is said to be stereospecific, if starting materials differ from its product only in the configuration.

Sterile water A form in which water is distributed in sterile packages and the sterile water for injection is intended mainly for use as a solvent for parenteral products.

Sterile water for inhalation It is water that is purified by distillation or by reverse osmosis and rendered sterile. It contains no antimicrobial agents, except where used in humidifiers or similar devices. This type of water should not be used for parenteral administration or for other sterile dosage forms.

Sterile water for injection It is water for injection that is sterilized and packaged in single-dose containers of type I and II glass. These containers do not exceed a capacity of 1 L. The limitations for total solids depend on the size of the container.

Sterilization The methed applied for destroying or removing of living cells, like viable spores, viruses, and viroids from an object or habitat.

Steroids A group of organic compounds with a nucleus of 17 carbon atoms as four fused rings (three containing six carbon atoms and one containing five) and with changeable substituents and degrees of unsaturation.

Sterols Terpenoids, solid, unsaturated steroid alcohols with an −OH group at the C3 position that occur both free and as esters or glycosides, and are classified according to the organism in which they occur as mycosterols, phytosterols, etc.

Sticking Sticking is adhesion of tablet material to a die wall. These problems are caused by excessive moisture or the inclusion of substances with low melting temperatures in the formulation.

Sticktight Nut that adheres firmly to shell after harvest.

Stigma Top tip/portion of the pistil of a flower usually located at the upper extremity of the style to get the pollen.

Stimulant A herb or drug that has the ability of exciting the activity of the body.

Stipe Also known as stalk.

Stipel The minute secondary stipule seen at the base of a leaflet.

Stipule One among the two membranaceous processes developed at base of a leaf petiole, either as tendril or as spine.

Stock Part of the root or stem to which the scion is variously attached or inserted during grafting.

Stoichiometry The study of the interaction between the amounts of product and the reactant.

Stolon Developing a new plant from the stem above the ground, with root at the tip.

Stoma (plural: stomata) The minute opening through which gaseous interchange between the atmosphere and the intercellular spaces within these structures occur. They are found in the epidermis of leaves, stems, and other plant organs and are associated with guard cells and accessory cells.

Stomachic An herb or agent that gives strength to stomach or motivate the appetite by increasing the digestive secretions.

Stoneworts A group of algae with a complex growth pattern, with nodal regions from which whorls of branches arise; they are plentiful in all fresh to brackish waters.

Strain A population of organisms that are isolated from either a single organism or a pure culture.

Stratified The periclinally running bands of fibers interspersed with the conducting tissue in phloem.

Streak plate A petri dish containing a solid culture medium prepared by spreading a microbial mixture over the agar surface, using an inoculating loop, the streak plate has the isolated microbial colonies growing on its surface.

Streptococcal pneumonia The endogenous infection in lungs caused by *Streptococcus pneumoniae* due to the predisposed individuals.

Streptococcal sore throat The common bacterial infections in humans caused by *Streptococcus* spp through the infected droplets of saliva or nasal secretions. It is also called as strep throat.

Striate Numerous parallel longitudinal lines or ridges, frequently rather fine and close and separated by groves.

Strobilus Firmly clustered group of sporophylls arranged on a central stalk; usually called a 'cone' or 'flower'.

Stroma Compact spore producing structure formed on the surface of a host by fungal mycelium.

Stromatolite Dome-shaped microbial mat communities having filamentous photosynthetic bacteria and occluded sediments, with a laminar structure.

Structural gene A gene that codes with a nonregulatory function to synthesis a polypeptide or polynucleotide.

Structure-activity relationship The relationship between chemical structure and pharmacological activity for a series of compounds.

Structure-based design The drug design approach based on the 3-D structure of the target obtained by X-ray or NMR.

Structure-property correlations All statistical mathematical scheme used to correlate the structural property to any other property either intrinsic, chemical or biological, by means of statistical regression and pattern recognition techniques.

Stub cotton The cotton crop where the stalks are cut down after harvest and the crown and rootstock are left in the ground for regrowth.

Style Slender upper portion of pistil, sustaining stigma.

Styloid Crystalline form of calcium oxalate with single elongated crystals that are pointed or square at the ends.

Styptic Any substance that can stops external bleeding.

Subacute cutaneous lupus erythematosus (SCLE) A form of non-scarring, photosensitive lupus skin disease, which can appear as red rings or as scaly plaques that can resemble psoriasis.

Subatomic particles The three kinds of particles, which make up atoms, i.e. protons, neutrons and electrons.

Subculture The aseptic transfer of a culture or a part of it to a fresh media.

Subcutaneous The fatty layer of tissue beneath the dermal part of the skin.

Subcutaneous injection The drug is injected beneath the skin.

Because the subcutaneous region is less vascular than muscle tissues, drug absorption is less rapid. The factors that affect absorption from intramuscular depots also affect subcutaneous absorption.

Suber Cork.

Suberin The waxy substance, formed in the corky cells of periderm layers that can resistant to microbial attack.

Suberization The formation of periderm layers on the cut surfaces or wounds of plants.

Subgingival plaque The plaque that forms at the dentogingival margin and extends down into the gingival tissue.

Sublimation The process of vaporizing a solid substance by heat.

Submerged plants Plants growing with their root, stems, and leaves completely under the surface of the water.

Subshrub Of habit, a low shrub, sometimes with partly herbaceous stems.

Subsidiary cells Epidermal cells that are clearly differentiated from the others and that immediately surround the guard cells of the stomata.

Sub-species A sub-division of species larger than a race.

Subsurface biosphere The region below the plant root zone where microbial populations can grow and function.

Subterranean Growing beneath the surface of the soil.

Subulate Narrow and tapering gradually to a fine point.

Successive cambia Refers to secondary thickening where a series of vascular cambia are initiated sequentially, each one cutting off phloem externally and xylem internally, as well as other tissues.

Succulent That which is full of juice or sap.

Succussion The process of powerfully arresting a homeopathic remedy against a firm surface.

Sucker Shoot occurring from the rootstock or trunk.

Sucrose Disaccharide consisting of glucose and fructose.

Sudorific The drug/herb adminstered internally, to promote sweating.

Suffrutescent The plant having a woody lower part and upper part is herbaceous.

Sugar and chocolate-coated tablets Sugar and chocolate-coated tablets are compressed tablets that are coated for various reasons. The coating may be added to protect the drug from air and humidity, to provide a barrier to a drug's objectionable taste or smell, or to improve the appearance of the tablet.

Sulfate reduction The method that involves the use of sulfate as an oxidizing agent, resulting to the accumulation of reduced forms of sulfur or incorporation of sulfur into organic molecules, usually as sulfhydryl groups.

Sulfide Any organic compound with sulfur bonded to the carbon.

Sulfoxide Any organic compound having the sulfur atom bonded to an oxygen.

Summer planting A scheme where planting is done in summer and fruits production begin in the following spring.

Summer wood It refers to late wood.

Sun checking Cracking of the entire kernels of grain due to the exposure to discontinuous conditions of dew, sun, and water stress.

Sun screen The products that blocks electromagnetic radiation (ultraviolet light) from entering the skin. Chemical sun screens can absorb ultraviolet energy while physical sun screens block or reflect UV radiation before it enters the skin.

Superantigen The bacterial proteins that can motivate the immune system more than the normal antigens.

Superinfection The new infection (bacterial or fungal) in a patient which are resistant to the drug(s) being used for treatment.

Superoxide dismutase An enzyme that catalyze the dismutation reaction of superoxide anion to dihydrogen peroxide and dioxygen to protects us by catalyzing the destruction of the toxic superoxide radical. They have active *sites* containing either copper and zinc (Cu/Zn-superoxide dismutase), or iron (Fe-superoxide dismutase), or manganese (Mn-superoxide dismutase).

Superposability The capability to fetch two particular stereochemical formulae into coincidence or to be superpose exactly in space, or to become accurate replicas of each other by no more than translation and rigid rotation.

Suppository Pharmaceutical preparation meant for inserting either into the rectum, vagina or urethra where it melts. After it is inserted, a suppository either melts at body temperature or dissolve (or disperses) into the aqueous secretion of the body cavity.

Suppressor mutation The mutation that conquers the effect of another mutation and produces the normal phenotype.

Surfactant Any substance that changes the nature of a surface, such as lowering the surface tension of water.

Suspended solids Undissolved solids, which can be removed by filtration.

Suspension A specific category of pharmaceutical product that must be in a colloidal dispersion (suspension) for proper action. It is a two-phase system that is composed of a solid material dispersed in an oily or aqueous liquid. The particle size of the dispersed solid is usually greater than 0.5 mm.

Suspension culture It is the system of single cells and small cell aggregates in a liquid growth medium. Process of agitation by bubbling, shaking or stirring is envolved to prevent settling of cells.

Suture The line of junction between two fused organs, occasionally also a line of dehiscence.

Svedberg unit The unit used in expressing the sedimentation coefficient; the greater a particle's Svedberg value, the faster it travels in a centrifuge.

Swab A wad of absorbent material usually wound around one end of a little stick and meant for applying medication or for removing material from a particular area.

Swainsonia Refers to polyhydroxy-alkaloid.

Swale The vacant or depression, particularly one in wet, muddy ground.

Swamp Spongy land or a low ground filled with water or a wooded area containing surface water almost all the time.

Swarm cell A flagellated cell or the motile cells of the Myxomycota.

Symbiosis The existing or close association of two unlike organisms.

Symbiosome The last nitrogen-fixing form of Rhizobium specifically active within root nodules.

Symmetry Representing the associations of the different parts of a structure about its axis.

Sympathetic system The subdivision of the autonomic nervous system, which dominates in stressful or emergency situations and prepares the body for strenuous physical activity.

Sympatric Distributions of two taxa, with similar ranges.

Sympetalous The petals when united by their margins or at least at the base.

Sympodial Growth of axillary shoots when apical budding has died down.

Symptom An alteration occurring during a disease, a person individually experiences, e.g. discomfort, pain, fatigue or loss of appetite).

Synangium Cluster of sporangia that got fused while developing.

Syncarp When the structure is made from several united fruits, generally fleshy.

Syncarpous Gynoecium containing two or more carpels, that is more or less congenitally fused together.

Synergy When two or more constituents work together to potentiate the effect or one constituent may modify the toxic effects of another (attenuating synergy); or when one constituent stabilizes or protects another (protective synergy).

Synonym The other names.

Synthase The enzyme that catalyzes the reaction to synthesise a particular molecule but not essentially through the formation of a bond between two molecules.

Syntrophism The involvement where an organism depends on, or is improved by the growth factors or nutrients by a neighboring organism. When both organisms benefit. Then it is called cross-feeding or the satellite phenomenon.

Syrups Syrups are traditionally peroral solutions that contain high concentrations of sucrose or other sugars. Through common usage, the term syrup has also come to include any other liquid dosage form prepared in a sweet, viscous vehicle.

Systemic The term defining the internal features of an illness, (e.g. kidney disease, heart disease, lung disease).

T

Tablet A powder with active substances and binders, pressed into a solid.

Tablet triturates Tablet triturates are small, usually cylindrical molded or compressed tablets. They are made of powders created by moistening the powder mixture with alcohol and water. They are used for compounding potent drugs in small doses.

Tangential flow filtration A separation technique employed for the transfer of components of one system (stream) into another.

Tannin They are complex mixture of polyphenols present in the bark of many shrubs and trees and precipitate proteins.

Taproot The large primary root which grows vertically downward and giving off small lateral roots.

Tautomerism Isomerism of the general form.

Tautomerization The isomerization by which tautomers are interconverted. It is a heterolytic molecular re-arrangement and is frequently very rapid.

Taxon A taxonomic category in which a group with related organisms are classified.

Taxonomic synonyms Taxonomically the name of a genus combined with a specific epithet.

Taxonomy The science that deals with the identification, nomenclature, and classification of objects of biological origin.

Tay-Sachs disease An inherited disease caused by a recessive gene mutation in infancy resulting in the profound mental retardation and early death.

TB skin test Carried out to detect the tuberculin hypersensitivity for a previous or current infection with *Mycobacterium tuberculosis*.

T cell (T lymphocyte) The blood cell that originates from bone marrow, but which matures in the thymus, of which some are responsible for cell-mediated immunity and production of antibodies.

T cell antigen receptor (TCR) The receptors on the T cell surface with two antigen-binding peptide chains and are associated with a large number of other glycoproteins.

T-dependent antigen The antigen that stimulates B cell response only in presence of T-helper cells that produce interleukin-2 and B cell growth factor.

Tegmen The part of the seed coat that develops from the inner integument.

Telophase The last stage of mitosis where the chromosomes get migrated to opposite poles and form a new nuclear envelope and then the chromosomes loosen.

Temperate phages Bacteriophages which infect the bacteria and create a lysogenic relationship slightly, than immediately lysing their hosts.

Temperature The specific degree of intensity of heat.

Template strand A strand of either DNA or RNA that identifies the basic sequence of a newly produced complementary strand of DNA or RNA.

Tendril These are slender twining, that are a modified form of stem or part of a leaf, to facilitate some plants climb.

Tensiometer The device used for measuring soil moisture, having a buried tube of water that builds up a partial vacuum as surrounding soil dries off.

Tepal When the sepals and petals of a flower are indistinguishable, they are referred to as tepals.

Teratogen A teratogen is a substance that produces a malformation in a foetus.

Terete Cylindrical or almost like it.

Terminal sterilization The process by which a non-sterile product is converted to a sterile one by sealing it in its final container.

Terminator A sequence where the transcription is stoped or the end of gene is marked.

Terpene It refers to any of several isomeric hydrocarbons.

Terrestrial The general habitat which is growing of or on the ground, e.g. plant growing on land.

Tertiary treatment The process that employs chemical and biological methods for the removal of inorganic nutrients, heavy metals, viruses, etc. from sewage, after microorganisms have been degraded during secondary sewage treatment.

Testa The outer covering or integument of seed, is hard.

Tetanolysin A hemolysin that aids in tissue destruction and is produced by *Clostridium tetani*.

Tetanospasmin The neurotoxic component of the tetanus toxin produced under the control of a plasmid gene resulting in muscle spasms of tetanus.

Tetanus Muscle spasms and convulsions caused by the anaerobic, spore-forming bacillus.

Tetracytic The stomata, surrounded by four subsidiary cells, of it two are parallel and the other two (often smaller) are at right angles to the long axis of the guard cells.

Tetrahydrofolates Tetrahydrofolates are referred to as the carriers of activated one carbon units that play an important part in the biosynthesis of amino acids and precursors needed for DNA synthesis, they reduce the folate derivatives that contain additional hydrogen atoms in positions 5, 6, 7 and 8.

Tetrapartite associations A mutualistic involvement of the identical plant with three different kind of microorganisms.

Thalassemia It is a chronic inherited disease resulting in the defective synthesis of hemoglobin, anemia that can be severe and is found more frequently in areas prone for malaria.

Thallophyta A primary division of plants with all forms consisting of one cell and cell aggregates not evidently differentiated into root, stem, and leaf, including bacteria, algae, fungi, and lichens.

Thallus Plant body that requires differentiation into separate forms of stems, leaves, roots, and does not grow from an apical point.

T-helper (TH) cell A cell that is needed for T cell-dependent antigens to be effectively presented to B cells, also, it promotes cell-mediated immune responses.

Theoretical yield The quantity that would be yielded at any suitable stage of manufacture, processing, or packing of a particular drug product, based on the quantity of components to be used, in the absence of any loss or error in actual production.

Therapeutic equivalent drug products Therapeutic equivalent drug products are pharmaceutical equivalents that can be expected to have the same clinical effect and safety profile when administered to patients under the same I' conditions specified in the labeling.

Therapeutic index It is the ratio between toxic and therapeutic doses or the ability of a substance to lessen disease, pain or injury (the higher the ratio, the greater the safety of the therapeutic dose).

Therapeutic touch It is a practise in which the registered or a practitioner assesses where a person's energy field is weak and congested and then uses his or her hands to direct energy into the field so as to balance it.

Thermal death time (TDT) The shortest period of time needed to kill all the organisms in a microbial population at a specified temperature and under defined conditions.

Thermodynamics The study that deals with heat and energy flow in chemical reactions.

Thermolysin It is the neutral protease isolated from aperticular bacteria and contains calcium- and zinc-containing.

Thermolysis An uncatalysed bond cleavage occurring due to the exposure of any compound to a heigher temperature.

Thermophile Any organism that could grow well at a temperature that is more than 50°C (122°F).

Therophytes The annual plants that overwinters as a seed.

Thigmotropism It is the directional growth response (tropism) which occurs in a plant or part of a plant to touch.

Thiosulfinate The organic compound with two sulfur atoms bonded together, of which one has a double bonded to an oxygen atom.

Thorax It refers to second among the three major divisions in the body of an insect with legs and wings.

Thorn It refers to a sharp rigid process on a plant.

Threatened species Any species of plant which is likely to become endangered if limiting factors are not reversed.

Three-dimensional quantitative structure-activity relationship The method of analyzing the quantitative relationship between the biological activity of a set of compounds and their spatial properties by means of statistical methods.

Thrombin (blood coagulation factor II) An enzyme (the activated thrombogen) formed in the blood, that can convert fibrinogen into fibrin for the formation of clot. It is formed from conjunction of prothrombin and calcium salts.

Thrombosis Clotting within a blood vessel that may cause infarction of tissues supplied by the vessel.

Thrush A disease observed in infants caused by parasitic fungus characterized by white specks inside the nose, throat, and mouth.

Thylakoid A flat sac found within the chloroplast stroma having photosynthetic pigments and the photosynthetic electron transport chain, it traps the light energy uses it in the form of ATP and NAD(P)H in the thylakoid membrane.

Thymine The pyrimidine 5-methyluracil which occurs in nucleosides, nucleotides, and DNA.

Thymol blue Thymolsulphonphthalein($C_{27}H_{30}O_5S$), is an acid-base indicator, which changes from pink to yellow as the pH is raised from 2.2 and then to blue as the pH is raised through 8.8.

Thymus It is a primary lymphoid organ present in the chest, and is required for the development of immunological functions and maturation of T cell.

Ti-plasmid A plasmid used to insert genes into plant cells, obtained from *Agrobacterium tumefaciens* that is.

Tiller The stem branches of a grass plant.

Tilosomes Refer to the masses of cellulosic and/or ligneous material in cells of the velamen next to the passage cells.

Tincture The medicine that containes a desired amount of glycerine, alcohol, or vinegar along with a herb, its prepared by soaking the herbs in a dark place with a solvent for 2 to 6 weeks.

Tincture of iodine The germicidal solution of iodine in aqueous alcohol used as an antiseptic on skin and tissue.

Tinea A name used for different kinds of superficial fungal infections of the skin, nails and hair, the specific type is (depending on characteristic appearance, etiologic agent, and site) generally designated by a modifying term.

Tinea capitis The fungal infection caused by species of Trichophyton or Microsporum on scalp hair.

Tinea cruris Also known as jock itch, a fungal infection of the groin caused by either *Epidermophyton floccosum*, *Trichophyton mentagrophytes* or *T. rubrum*.

Tinea manuum The fungal infection caused by *Trichophyton rubrum*, *T. mentagrophytes*, or *E. floccosum* on hands.

Tinea pedis The fungal infection caused by *Trichophyton rubrum*, *T. mentagrophytes*, or *E. floccosum* on the foot so its also known as athlete's foot.

Tinea unguium The fungal infection caused by either *Trichophyton rubrum or T. mentagrophytes* on the nailbed.

Tissue The functional unit of protein molecules. A group of tissue form an organ, e.g. kidney, brain or heart.

Tissue culture The process by which a mass of cells (callus) is produced from an explant, and the callus produced could be directly used either to regenerate plantlets or to either primary or secondary metabolites.

Titer (the amount of sample) The strength of a solution or the concentration of a substance in solution as determined by titration.

Titration Volumetric analysis in which a definite amounts of a test solution is added to solution containing a known amount of the substance analyzed.

Tolerance Refers to the failure to mount an immune reaction on exposure to what would normally be an antigenic substance.

Tolerance level Highest percentage of a disease or pest symptom that could be allowed during field inspections for certification of a seed lot; levels are different with each field generation and can vary in individual state.

Tonic Any herb or substance that strengthens the system, tonics can be a stimulants or alternatives.

Tonsillitis The inflammation of the tonsils.

Top crop The fruits that are formed in the second fruiting cycle of cotton, mostly on upper branches.

Topical product A pharmaceutical products that can be applied to the skin or soft tissue in the form of liquid, cream, or ointment.

Topliss tree It is an operational scheme for the design of analog.

Topoisomerase 1 antibody It is an autoantibody seen in the blood of patients suffering from systemic sclerosis.

Topomerisation The identity reaction which results in the exchange of the positions of an identical ligands. The indistinguishable molecular entities involved are called topomers.

Tortuous Any thing that is irregular and more or less spirally twisted.

Total bacteria count The evaluation of the total number of bacteria in a sample based on standard methods procedures for collecting, incubating, and counting colony-forming units.

Total body clearance Total body clearance is the drug elimination rate divided by the plasma drug concentration.

Total dissolved solids (TDS) The term used to describe inorganic ions in the water. Usually measured by electrical conductance of the water corrected to 25°C, and expressed as ppm (parts per million).

Total heat (TH) The total of sensible heat and latent heat.

Total ionized solids Concentration of dissolved ions in solution expressed in concentration units of sodium chloride (NaCl). It determines the operating life of ion exchange resins and is calculated from measurements of specific resistance.

Total organic carbon (TOC) It is a parameter in determining the purity of semiconductor grade water, in which the measure of level of organic impurities in water by their carbon content that concludes the operating life of activated carbon beds.

Total solids Total solids is the measure of both dissolved and suspended solids in water established by weighing sample before and after evaporation.

Totipotency The ability of plant cells to regenerate into a whole plants when cultured on appropriate medium.

Toxemia The condition produced by toxins in the blood of any host.

Toxic It refers to a substance that is harmful.

Toxic shock-like syndrome (TSLS) A disease produced by an invasive group. For example, the infections caused by *Streptococcus* are characterized by a rapid drop in blood pressure, failure of different organs, and a very high fever due to the release of streptococcal pyrogenic exotoxins.

Toxic shock syndrome A type of staphylococcal disease, commonly seen in females who make use of certain types of tampons during menstruation caused due to the production of toxic shock syndrome toxin by certain strains of *Staphylococcus aureus*.

Toxicity Any drug with a poisonous nature to the body.

Toxicokinetics Toxicokinetics is the application of pharmacokinetic principles to the design, conduct and interpretation of drug safety evaluation studies.

Toxicology A science that involves in the study of the effects, and the problems associated with poisons.

Toxigenicity The ability of an organism to produce a toxin.

Toxin A microbial product which could injure another cell or organism at a very low concentrations. They are commonly the poisonous protein, but some times lipids and other substances.

Toxin neutralization The process involved in the inactivation of toxins by specific antibodies, called antitoxins.

Toxoid A bacterial exotoxin which is modified, so that it is no longer toxic in nature but will stimulate the formation of antitoxin when injected into a person or animal.

Toxoplasmosis The disease caused by the parasitic protozoan (*Toxoplasma gondii*) in both animals and human being.

Trace analysis It is the analysis of any constituents in ppm and ppb concentrations. Ultrapure type I reagent grade water and extremely pure reagents have been used for the estimation.

Trace elements Elements required for physiological functions at very small concentration, that vary for different organisms. Examples include Co, Cu, F, Fe, I, Mn, Mo, Ni, Se, V, W and Zn.

Tracer A radioactive isotope is one which is incorporated into a compound of biological importance so as to find the pathway through the physiological processes of the plant.

Tracheary tissue It is a common term used for tissues or elements made of tracheary elements, e.g. xylem, tracheids and vessel members.

Tracheid Tracheids are capillary tube produced from a sequence of dead cells in the xylem, or a single such cell, where at least the middle lamella of the end walls remains intact.

Tracheophyta The group of plants consisting of green plants with a vascular system that includes tracheids or tracheary elements, being the Pteridophyta and Spermatophyta, commonly called vascular plants.

Trachoma A chronic infectious disease of the conjunctiva and cornea, resulting in pain, inflammation and occasionally blindness. Caused by *Chlamydia trachomatis serotypes* A-C.

Transamination The process of removal of amino group from an amino acid by transferring it to an α-keto acid acceptor.

Transcriptase The enzyme that catalyzes transcription; in viruses with RNA genomes, the enzyme is RNA-dependent. RNA polymerase that is used to make RNA copies of the RNA genomes.

Transcription The genetic information encoded in the gene, is copied into an exactly complementary sequence of ribonucleotides known as mRNA (messenger RNA).

Transdermal Transdermal (percutaneous) drug absorption is the placement of the drug (in a lotion, ointment, cream, paste, or patch) on the skin surface for systemic absorption.

Transdermal patch The adhesive patch (medicated) that is placed on the skin to release timely dose of medication through the skin and into the bloodstream.

Transduction The transfer of genetic informations from one cell to another by means of a viral vector (for bacteria, the vector is Bacteriophage).

Transfection The acquirement of new genetic markers by addition of viral DNA to cells.

Transfer RNA (tRNA) A type of RNA with triplet nucleotide sequences that are complementary to the triplet nucleotide coding sequences of mRNA. They bond with amino acids and transfer them to the ribosomes during the protein synthesis, where proteins are assembled according to the genetic code.

Transferase The enzyme, which help in the catalysis of opne group from one substrate to another.

Transferrin The iron-transport protein of blood plasma, that has two similar iron-binding domains with high affinity for Fe(III).

Transformation A mode of gene transfer in bacteria in which a piece of free DNA is taken up by a bacterial cell and integrated into the recipient genome.

Transformation products Chemicals derived from particular compound, during extraction, processing, or spontaneous decomposition.

Transgenic animal or plant An animal or plant that has gained new genetic information from the inclusion of foreign DNA. Like injection of DNA into animal eggs, electroporation of mammalian cells and plant cell protoplasts,

Transition mutations Mutations that involve the substitution of a different purine base for the purine present at the site of the mutation or the substitution of a different pyrimidine for the normal pyrimidine.

Translation It is the process involved in the protein synthesis where the genetic message carrier the mRNA directs the synthesis of polypeptides with the aid of ribosomes and other cell constituents.

Translocated herbicide That which has the ability to move throughout a plant after being applied to leaf surfaces.

Translucent One which is transmitting light or transparent.

Transmission electron microscope The microscope involves the principle of forming the image by passing an electron beam through a specimen and focusing the scattered electrons with magnetic lenses.

Transpiration The process in which the water vapor is evaporated from plants, generally through a stomata.

Transversion mutations Mutations which occurs due to the substitution of either a purine base for the normal pyrimidine or a pyrimidine for the normal purine.

Trap crop Either a crop or a segment of a crop planned to attract pests so that they can be destroyed by treating a small area or by destroying the trap crop along with the pests together.

Traveler's diarrhea A form of diarrhea caused because of the ingestion of certain viruses, bacteria, or protozoa normally absent from the traveler's environment.

Treatment investigational new drug Investigational new drug formulates promising new drug available to those patients who are desperately ill. FDA permits the drug to be used if there is preliminary evidence of efficacy and it treats a serious or life-threatening disease, or if there is not comparable therapy available.

Treatment threshold The level of pest population at which a pesticide or other control measures are required to avoid eventual financial injury to the crop.

Tree A tall plant, it could be either a conifers, flowering plants or extinct lycophytes and sphenophytes.

Tremor The involuntary movement that occurs in part or parts of the body.

Tricarboxylic acid cycle (TCA) The cycle, which oxidizes acetyl coenzyme A to CO_2 and generates NADH and $FADH_2$ for oxidation in the electron transport chain. This cycle also supplies carbon skeletons for biosynthesis.

Trichome Also known as hairs or scales, that outgrowth of the epidermis, or a row or filament of bacterial cells that are in close contact with each another over a large area.

Trichomoniasis It is a sexually transmitted disease which is caused by the parasitic protozoan *Trichomonas vaginalis*.

Trichoscleried It is long slender sclereid cell generally with branches.

Trichotomous That which branches equally or almost equally into three parts.

Trickling filter The bed of rocks roofed with a microbial film which aerobically degrades organic waste during the treatment of secondary sewage.

Trifid One which is deeply divided into three parts.

Trifoliolate With three leaflets.

Triglyceride A compound consisting of three fatty acids along with glycerol.

Trinucleate The pollen grains in which the male gametophyte has three nuclei when it is shed from the anther.

Tripinnate The leaf which is thrice pinnately divided.

Triploid Having the chromosome number that is three times the monoploid number.

Tristichous That which is arranged in three vertical rows.

Triterpenoids The largest single class of terpenoids with six isoprene units as their basic structure.

Tropane It is the basic unit of tropane alkaloids, ornithine as an intermediate and is a bicyclic compound.

Trophozoite The active/motile feeding stage of protozoan organism; as in malarial parasite, the stage of schizogony between the ring stage and the schizont.

Tropism The movement of living organisms either in the direction of or away from a focus of heat, light, or other stimulus.

Tropophyll Leaf that serves for assimilation.

True leaf The leaf which is produced after the cotyledons.

True pollen Refers to the microspore having distal rather than proximal germination and no marks where the grains were attached to each other in the tetrad.

Truncate Mainly of leaves (shapes), terminating abruptly, as if tapering end were cut off; cut squarely across, either at the base or apex of an organ.

Trunk The main stem of a tree, except its roots and branches.

Trypanosome Trypanosomes are parasitic flagellate protozoa that often live in the blood of humans and other vertebrates and are transmitted by insect bites, they belong to genus Trypanosoma.

Trypanosomiasis An infection caused due to trypanosomes that live in the blood and lymph of the infected host.

Tuber The modified form of underground stem, that provides storage of nutrients, e.g. potato.

Tubercle The small root swelling or nodule, a surficial nodule; a thickened, solid, spongy crown or cap, as on an achene; a small tuber or tuber-like growth.

Tuberculoid (neural) leprosy A type of leprosy that is gentle and nonprogressive, it is associated with delayed-type hypersensitivity to antigens on the surface of

Mycobacterium leprae and also early nerve damage along with regions of skin that have lost sensation and are surrounded by a border of nodules.

Tuberculosis An infectious disease caused by Mycobacterium in humans and other animals and is characterized by the formation of tubercles and tissue necrosis, primarily as a result of host hypersensitivity and inflammation.

Tuberculous cavity It is the cavity filled with air caused due to tubercle lesion by *M. tuberculosis*.

Tuberization Formation of tubers at the ends of stolons; tuber initiation.

Tumid One which is swollen or inflated.

Tumor The abnormal growth of cells.

Tumor inducing principle Refers to a plasmid, which is carried by bacterium *Agrobacterium tumefaciens* that causes crown gall disease in plants. The plasmid is essential for converting normal tissue of host into tumour tissue which involves incorporation of plasmid into the plant genome. Most interestingly the tissue removed from crown gall tumours can grow in culture medium without adding auxin and cytokinin.

Tumor necrosis factor Tumor necrosis factor is a lymphokine produced by macrophages. It can be activated to kill tumor cells.

Tumor pathogenesis It is the morphological and physiological changes caused during tumor growth.

Tunic Specially of a corm or bulb, a thin membranous or fibrous outer covering.

Turbidity It is a suspension of fine particles that obscures light rays but requires many days for sedimentation because of small particle size.

Turbidostat It is the continuous culture system that is operational with a photocell that adjusts the flow of medium through the culture vessel so as to maintain a constant cell density or turbidity.

Turbinate Shape of a cone while resting on its apex.

Turgid Swollen due to high water content.

Twig The tiny shoot or branch of a tree or plant.

Type I hypersensitivity A type of immediate hypersensitivity occurring due the binding of antigen to IgE attached to mast cells, which will release anaphylaxis mediators such as histamine, e.g. hay fever, asthma, and food allergies.

Type II hypersensitivity A type of immediate hypersensitivity in which the binding of antibodies to antigens on cell surfaces is followed by destruction of the target cells (e.g. through complement attack, phagocytosis, or agglutination).

Type III hypersensitivity A type of immediate hypersensitivity occurring due to the excess exposure to antigens in which antibodies bind to the antigens and produce antibody-antigen complexes. It activates the complement and triggers an acute inflammatory response with subsequent tissue damage, e.g. serum sickness.

Type IV hypersensitivity It is the delayed hypersensitivity response, which appears after 24 to 48 hours after the exposure to antigen. It results from the binding of antigen to activated T lymphocytes, which later on release cytokines and trigger inflammation and macrophage attacks that damage tissue. Type IV hypersensitivity is seen in contact dermatitis from poison ivy, leprosy, and tertiary syphilis.

Tyrosine (Tyr) Phenolic alpha amino acid. It acts as a precursor of hormones, epinephrine, norepinephrine, thyroxine, and triiodothyronine, and of the black pigment melanin.

U

Ulcer Internal sore that is open.

Ultracentrifugation The method of separation of macromolecules on the basis of their density and shape using the gravitational field generated in a high-speed centrifuge.

Ultrafiltration It is a membrane pores very small enough to remove large molecules. Rated in terms of nominal molecular weight cutoff. A 10,000 Dalton (molecular weight) UF membrane, e.g. will remove bacterial pyrogens that are typically in the range of 20,000 Daltons.

Ultrafine particle Refers to particle with an equivalent diameter less than 0.1 µm.

Ultra low penetration air (ULPA) filters Refer to extended media dry filters in a rigid frame, which have a minimum particle-collection efficiency of 99.999% for particles greater than or equal to 0.12 µm in size, commonly used in microelectronics and in pharmaceuticals.

Ultramicrobacteria A bacteria that can or is capable to exist normally in a miniaturized form in low-nutrient conditions. They may be 0.2 mm or more smaller.

Ultrapure water The water with a specific resistance greater than 1 megohm-cm, also referred as type I reagent grade water in laboratory.

Ultraviolet oxidation UV radiation is employed in purification of water for the photochemical oxidation of organic impurities so as to get HPLC grade water with very low level of organic impurity (i.e. less than 0.0005 absorbance units).

Ultraviolet (UV) radiation It is of fairly short wavelength, (200 to 400 nm), and high energy.

Ultraviolet sterilizer Ultraviolet lamps that can kill microorganisms present in water.

Ultraviolet TOC reduction An ultraviolet source, which partially oxidizes organic compounds to ionic species, which can be removed. It relies on 185 nm (nanometer) radiation from ozone producing mercury lamps, along with 254 nm germicidal radiation.

Umbel Raceme inflorescence in which all the individual flower stalks arising in a cluster at the top of the peduncle and are of equal length.

Umbellate Forming an umbel or umbels.

Umbelliferone A coumarin.

Uncinate That which finishes in a hooked point.

Undulate The margin of leaf blade, with vertical undulations, not essentially to have a teeth.

Unfurled Unopened.

Uni (prefix) One of whatever is qualified.

Uniaxial With axis composed of one single filament.

Unicellular Any thing with only a single cell.

Unidirectional airflow Earlier known as laminar airflow. It is the rectified airflow through the entire cross-section of a clean zone with a steady velocity. This results in a directed transport of particles from the clean zone.

Unifacial Normally in leaves, rounded or terete, without either adaxial or the abaxial surfaces.

Unifoliolate Refers to leaves, with compound leaves, but reduced to only one leaflet in this case, there being some sort of pulvinus or articulation at the apex of the petiole.

Uniform mechanical code The document with complete set of requirements for the design, construction, installation, and maintenance of heating, ventilating, cooling and refrigeration systems; incinerators and other heat-producing appliances.

Unilateral With reference to stamens, with anthers grouped on one side of the style.

Unilocular It refers to having only one internal cavity of an ovary/anther or fruit.

Unisexual Having either male or female reproductive organs, used for the gametophyte only.

Unit dose drug dispensing It is a technology that allocate all medications to the clinical unit in individual packages that recognize its name and dose. Unit-dose packaging is a key safety mea-

sure that facilitate to reduce the risk of drug distribution errors.

Universal precautions Precautions taken while handling, storing, transporting, or shipping the products or specimens either containing or are contaminated with human blood and body fluids: all such materials are treated as infectious.

Unsaturated fatty acid A fatty acid with one or more double bonds.

Uracil A pyrimidine 2,4-dioxypyrimidine, found in nucleotides, nucleosides and RNA, with a capability of forming a base pair with adenine.

Urease Urea amidohydrolase (nickel enzyme) that catalyzes the hydrolysis of urea to carbon dioxide and ammonia.

Urinalysis A test performed in urine to spot evidence of kidney disease or infection.

Urinary tract The passageways that facilitate the flow of urine, it starts in the kidney and takes it outside the body.

Urticarial vasculitis Blood vessel inflammation in the dermal part of the skin, with skin changes that look like hives.

USP (United States Pharmacopeia) It refers to the compendium of testing and purity criteria for pharmaceuticals, ancillaries, and raw materials.

Urushiol It is an oily, phenolic liquid obtained from plant source that cause severe skin irritation.

V

Vaccine It is a microbial preparation containing antigens that provoke the production of antibodies on injection, thus conferring immunity on the recipient. Vaccines are of three types. Those with a modified toxoid which had lost its toxic properties but retain its immunogenicity; one with live, attenuated organisms like virus or bacterium, and are antigenically similar to the original strain but lack virulence and those having material from a nonvirulent organism that retains its immunogenicity but does not result in infection.

Vacuoles These are membrane-bound organelles with low density responsible for food digestion, osmotic regulation, and waste product storage. They occupy up to 90% fraction of cell volume.

Vacuum degasification The process involved in removing of dissolved and entrained gases from the reverse osmosis (RO) product water by means of creating a vacuum in a tower through which this water flows.

Valence Maximum number of univalent atoms that facilitate to combine with an atom of the element under consideration or for which an atom of this element can be substituted.

Valence electrons Electrons present in the outermost shell of an atom.

Validation Any program that is documented and can provide assurance that a specific process, or system will over and over again produce a result meeting pre-determined acceptance criteria.

Validation master plan The standard plan for qualification of a facility or part of a facility, which identifies the layout of the operation, the associated utilities and systems, the equipment, and the processes to be validated. It also provides preliminary information as to the extent of the qualification and validation (IQ, OQ, PQ), required documentation, SOPs, acceptance criteria and responsibilities. It should also establish the cross reference of qualification projects by product, system, discipline, etc.

Validation protocol Any written plan/process, which can explain the process to be authenticated, including production equipment and how validation will be conducted. Such a plan would address objective test parameters, product and process characteristics, predetermined specifications, and factors that will determine acceptable results.

Valpotriates Category of iridoid monoterpenes, triesters of poly-alcohols with an iridoid structure and an epoxy group.

Valvate It is an aestivation, parts meeting edge to edge in the bud, neither overlapping or turned in one direction or another.

Valve When considered to an organ it is a part which has fragmented; while in a capsule, it is the portions into which the pericarp splits when mature.

van der Waals equation It is an equation intended for non-ideal gasses that accounts for intermolecular attraction and the volumes occupied by the gas molecules.

van der Waals force The attractive or repulsive forces between molecular entities (or between groups within the same molecular entity) other than those due to bond formation or to the electrostatic interaction of ions or of ionic groups with one another or with neutral molecules.

Vapor pressure Dalton's law for a mixture of perfect gases states that the mixture pressure is equivalent to the total of the partial pressures of the constituents. The partial pressure of moisture is called vapor pressure, and is expressed as,

Total pressure (Pt) = Partial pressure of air (Pa) + Partial pressure of moisture (Pv).

Varicose veins A condition in which the swollen veins are characterized by blue color, dilation, knotty appearance, and location close to surface of skin.

Variety A term sometimes used synonymously with cultivar, a taxonomic group below the species used in different senses by different specialists, usually referring to a strain which arises in nature as opposed to a cultivar which is specifically bred for particular properties.

Vascular bundle These are a group of specialized cells consisting of xylem and phloem, sometimes divided by a strip of cambium and arranged in different patterns.

Vascular cambium It is located between the xylem and phloem and is the lateral meristem that forms the secondary tissue.

Vascular system The plant tissues system that conducts water, mineral nutrients, and products of photosynthesis through the plant, it consists of xylem and phloem.

Vascular targeting agents (VTAs) The multifunctional agents that are home to the capillaries and vessels of solid tumors.

Vascular tissues They are conducting tissues made up of xylem and phloem.

Vasculitis Inflammatory injury that occurs on the blood vessels in the skin and other tissues. Usually the vasculitis lesions on the skin appear as purple spots on the legs.

Vasopermeation enhancement agents (VEAs) A new generation of drugs, which increase the uptake of therapeutic agents to solid tumors.

Vector An agent, (insect), that can carry a disease-producing organism from one host to another.

Vegetable alkali Generally crude or purified potassium carbonate (K_2CO_3).

Vegetative cell The male gametophyte of angiosperms that do not divide further.

Vegetative growth Without sexual reproduction or by cell divission.

Vehicle Any solvent or carrier fluid used in a pharmaceutical product with no pharmacological role, e.g. petroleum ether, chloroform, ethanol.

Vein The strand of vascular tissue.

Velocity The speed of an object; the change in position over time.

Venation It refers to the arrangement and pattern of veins in a leaf.

Venereal syphilis It is sexually transmitted disease caused by the spirochete *Treponema pallidum* and is contagious.

Verbascoside A phenylpropanoid, an ester of caffeic acid.

Vermicide The herb that kills intestinal worms.

Vermifuge Any herb or substance/drug that can expel or destroy intestinal worms.

Vernal Any thing that belongs to spring season.

Vernicose Varnished, as if the surface was varnished.

Verrucae vulgaris The raised, epidermal lesion with horny surface caused by an infection with a human papillomavirus.

Verrucose One with little warts or wart-like growth on the surface.

Versatile That which turns freely on its support.

Vertebrae The segments of the spinal column that is separated by disks made of connective tissue.

Vertebrate Any animal having a segmented vertebral column that include reptiles, mammals and birds.

Vertigo The condition distinguished by feelings of spinning of outside objects or self, dizziness, lost equilibrium, or giddiness.

Vesicant The agent that causes blistering, e.g. poison ivy.

Vesicle Any small bladder-like structure, cavity, sac, or cyst; with air filled.

Vesicular transport Vesicular transport is the process of engulfing particles or dissolved materials by a cell. Vesicular transport is the only transport mechanism that does not require a drug to be in an aqueous, solution to be absorbed. Pinocytosis and phagocytosis are forms of vesicular transport.

Vessel The capillary tube created from a series of dead cells, in xylem, the end walls are broken down entirely or partially and form scalariform or simple perforation plates.

Vestigial One which is reduced from the ancestral condition and does not work any more.

Veterinary Refers to pharmaceuticals or biologicals proposed for animal use.

Viable That which is capable of living and reproducing.

Vial A container usually of class I borosilicate glass for a parenteral product. Sealed with a rubber closure and over-seal.

Vibrio A bacterial cell, which is rod-shaped and is curved to form a comma or an incomplete spiral.

Vigor It is the capability of a plant for active vegetative growth.

Villous Pubescent, shaggy, covered with fine long hairs, but the hairs not matted.

Viroid The segment of infectious nucleic acid, with no protein coat of a virus.

Viral antigens A particular proteins on the capsid of a virus which could act as inducers of antibody formation.

Viral hemagglutination The process in which the viruses cause the clumping or agglutination of red blood cells.

Viral neutralization It is an antibody-mediated method in which IgA, IgM, and IgA antibodies bind to viruses during their extracellular phase and inactivate or neutralize them.

Viremia The occurrence of viruses in the bloodstream.

Viricide The agent that inactivates viruses so that the viruses cannot reproduce within host cells.

Virion A fully developed virus. Infection is initiated in a cell by a virion.

Virioplankton Viruses that are found in waters; high levels are found in marine and freshwater environments.

Viroid It is an infectious agent of plants with a single-strand of RNA, which is neither associated with any protein, nore codes for any proteins and is not translated.

Virology The division of microbiology which is concerned with viruses and viral diseases.

Virucide The agent that destroys or inactivates the viruses.

Virulence A disease-producing power of a microorganism.

Virulence factor Any bacterial product, generally a protein or carbohydrate, that contributes to virulence or pathogenicity.

Virus A noncellular parasite which can reproduce only inside living cells.

Viscid It is a thicky, syrupy, and sticky, viscous; covered with a viscid substance as of leaves.

Viscin threads These are very fine threads made up of material of

origin, connected to pollen grains and causing them to clump together when removed by the pollinator.

Viscosity The affinity of a liquid to oppose flowing because of molecular attraction (cohesion).

Viscous It refers to nature of a liquid, not pouring freely, having the consistency of syrup or honey.

Vital force It is the energy that maintains life in the individual.

Vitamin A group of organic substances, with a known or unknown composition, and present in minute amount in natural foodstuffs which are essential to normal metabolism. They are classified into two groups, the fat-soluble, and the water-soluble. Vitamins A, D, E, and K are fat-soluble. Vitamin C and members of the vitamin B complex group are water-soluble.

Vittae The sacs or tubes containing oil, e.g. in many fruits.

Vochysine The pyrrolidine alkaloid.

Volatile alkali It refers to aqueous ammonia, NH_3.

Volatile oil Also known as essential oil; they are odorous plant oil that evaporates readily.

Volatile Any substance that evaporates easily is assumed to be 'volatile'. Anything with a strong aroma is usually volatile, as the molecules can easily pass into the surrounding air.

Volume It measures the size of an object with the help of length measurements in three dimensions.

VPHP The microbiode contamination technology employed to decontaminate the exposed, internal surfaces within a sealed isolator and the exposed, external surfaces of materials and components placed within the sealed isolator. The process has four phases: a. Dehumidification, b. Conditioning (VPHP) at or below saturation conditions, c. Sterilization (VPHP) at or below saturation conditions, d. Aeration.

Wastewater treatment The employment of physical and biological processes to remove particulate and dissolved material from sewage and to control the pathogens.

Water activity The quantitative determination of water availability in the habitat; the water activity of a solution is one-hundredth its relative humidity.

Water for injection, USP The water purified by distillation or by reverse osmosis, with no added substance. It conforms to the standards of purified water, but is also free of pyrogen. It is used as a solvent for the preparation of parenteral solutions.

Water mold The universal term for a member of the division Oomycota.

Water treatment The water treatment is referred to as water conditioning, which consists of adding or removing of any chemical or chemicals to modify the properties of water.

Wave The signal that propagates through space.

Wavelength The length between two consecutive (low points) troughs or peaks (high points).

Waxes Substances which contain saturated and unsaturated hydrocarbons along with some substitution by oxygen.

Weak acid Any substance which cannot completely ionize in solution but is capable of donating hydrogen.

Weak bases Substances capable of accepting hydrogen.

Weakness The feeling of tiredness or muscle fatigue.

Weed Any wild plant that is of no use to man which makes its way into farm and gardens where it is not wanted.

Weil-Felix reaction The diagnosis of typhus and certain other rickettsial diseases.

Well-established-use product Any medicinal product that has established a firm reputation of quality, safety and efficacy through at least 10 years of regular, documented therapeutic use in the European Union.

Western blot The process by which a mixture of proteins is separated on a polyacrylamide gel and then transferred to a nylon membrane. The membrane can then be treated with reagents like specific antibodies to trace the protein of interest.

Wet weight Weight of plants after the outer surface covering of water has been removed. It is not a reliable measurement as this method in preparing the plants prior to weighing vary considerably.

Wet woodland The wooded area containing surface water for intermittent short periods.

White blood cell The blood cell without respiratory pigment. In vertebrates, it may be lymphocyte, polymorphonuclear leukocyte, or monocyte.

White piedra The fungal infection caused by *Trichosporon beigelii* (yeast) that forms light-colored nodules on the beard and mustache.

White roots These are secondary roots.

WHO World Health Organization

WHO guidelines for herbal medicines To describe basic criteria for the evaluation of quality, safety and efficacy of herbal medicines and thereby to assist national regulatory authorities, scientific organizations, and manufacturers to undertake an assessment of the documentation in respect of such products.

Whole-organism vaccine The vaccine made from complete pathogens, which are commonly of four types, like inactivated viruses; attenuated viruses; killed microorganisms; and live, attenuated microorganisms.

Whorl The display of appendages, for example branches or leaves, which are equally spaced around the stem at the same point, like the ribs of an umbrella.

Widal test A test involving agglutination of typhoid bacilli which when mixed with serum having typhoid antibodies from an individual having typhoid fever; for spoting the presence of *Salmonella typhi* and *S. paratyphi*.

Widebandtracheid A type of tracheid with tall wall thickenings and partially occluding the lumen.

Wighteone It is an isoflavone.

Wild type The most commonly encountered genotype in natural breeding populations.

Wilson's disease An inherited condition in which copper fails to be excreted in the bile. Copper accumulates progressively in the liver, brain, kidney and red blood cells. As the amount of copper accumulates hemolytic anaemia, chronic liver disease and a neurologic syndrome develop.

Wilt A plant which is bent towards the ground due to lack of water or heat.

Windowpane Removal of epidermal layer of a leaf tissue leaving small pieces of clear tissue.

Winter planting It is a method of planting in mid to late fall that depends on growth during winter months for the production of early spring crop.

Withanolides It is a steroidal lactones characterized by ergostane type steroids with C_{28} basic skeleton and has C_9 units a side chain of which a six-membered lactone ring is a characteristic feature.

Wood Any secondary tissue present in seed plants that is largely consisting of xylem tissue.

Woody Any substance which is made of or contain wood or wood fibers (mainly of hard lignified tissues).

Worms They are one of one hundred species of intestinal parasites with soft, long, rounded body and no legs or backbone.

Wort It is a filtrate of malted grain used as the substrate for the manufacture of beer and ale by the process of fermentation.

WTO World Trade Organisation.

X

X chromosome The sex chromosome that usually occurs paired in each female cell and single in each male cell in species in which the male typically has two unlike cell chromosomes.

Xanthones These are flavanone derivatives, derived from shikimic acid pathways or polyketides and combined with acetate-malonate units.

Xanthophylls Carotenoids which are oxygenated derivatives of simple unsaturated hydrocarbons.

Xanthosis It is a group of symptom with distorted leaf growth and yellow leaf margins which occurs in plants infected by mottle virus and either crinkle virus or mild yellow edge virus.

Xenobiotics It is an industrial chemicals with a chemical structure which is not found in natural compounds that could resist degradation by microorganisms.

Xenogamy Means cross-pollination, pollination of one plant by another.

Xeric It is characterized by a inadequate supply of moisture, tolerating, or adapted to arid environment.

Xeromorphic It is a structural feature associated with plants of arid habitats (e.g. hard or succulent leaves), even if the plant is not necessarily drought tolerant.

Xerophyte The plant which can tolerate drought.

Xerosis Another term denoting dry skin.

Xerotic eczema Severe dryness of the skin which leads to red irritable skin.

XPS (X-ray photoelectron spectroscopy) or ESCA (electron spectroscopy for chemical analysis) A surface-sensitive technique capable of detecting all elements with an atomic number greater than that of helium. ESCA provides data on the outermost several atomic layers of a material, and has a sensitivity in the order of 0.5 atomic percent. A primary advantage of ESCA is that it can both determine and quantify the chemical state of the elements detected, i.e. metallic state or oxide state.

Xylans It is a polysaccharide component of hemicellulose with xylose molecules.

Xylem It acts as supporting tissue and as water transporting system in plants. It consists of lignified tracheids or vessels.

Xylem parenchyma The parenchyma present in the wood.

Xylenol blue An acid-base indicator (chemically: 1,4-dimethyl-5-hydroxybenzenesulfonphthalein) which changes from red to yellow when the pH is raised from 2 and then to blue when the pH is raised through 8.8.

Xyloglucans It is a polysaccharide which is a component of hemicelluloses and contains molecules of both xylose and glucose.

Xylose It is a five carbon sugar (pentose) (CH_2OH $(CHOH)_3$ $CH=O$).

Y

Y chromosome The sex chromosome which is characteristic of male zygotes in species in which the male typically has two dissimilar sex chromosomes.

Yeast A unicellular fungus with a single nucleus and reproduces either by asexually (budding or fission), or sexually through spore formation.

Yeast artificial chromosome (YAC) A stretch of DNA that contains all the elements necessary to propagate a chromosome in yeast and which is used to clone foreign DNA fragments in yeast cells.

Yellow fever An acute infectious disease transmitted to humans by mosquitoes caused by a flavivirus.

Yield, expected The quantity of material or the percentage of theoretical yield anticipated at any appropriate phase of production based on previous laboratory or manufacturing data.

Yield, theoretical The quantity that would be produced at any suitable phase of manufacture, processing, or packing of a particular active pharmaceutical ingredient or intermediate, based upon the amount of components to be used, in the absence of any loss or error in actual production.

YM shift The change in shape by dimorphic fungi when they shift from the yeast (Y) form in the animal body to the mold or mycelial form (M) in the environment.

Yoga It is a posturing and breathing technique to stimulate relaxation.

Z

Z value The raise in temperature essential to decrease the decimal reduction time to one-tenth of its original value.

Zeatin It is a growth harmone which was first isolated from maize kernels and is a derivative of adenine.

Zeolite It is an hydrated alkali-aluminum silicate of either natural or synthetic origin which exhibits limited base exchange and is used as an ion exchange medium for the softening of hard water.

Zeta potential The positive charge or potential existing at the surface of a particle across the pH range.

Zone of differentiation Region of plant root where newly produced cells develop into different cell types.

Zone of elongation Region in plant root where newly produced cells grow and elongate just before differentiation.

Zoochory Spreading of diaspores by means of animals.

Zooflagellates Flagellate protozoa without chlorophyll which are either holozoic, symbiotic, or saprozoic.

Zoonosis It is a disease of animals which can be spread to humans.

Zooplankton A group of floating, aquatic, minute animals and nonphotosynthetic protists.

Zoospore It is a motile, flagellated spore.

Zooxanthella A dinoflagellate found living symbiotically within cnidarians and other invertebrates.

Zwitterionic compound Any neutral compound containing electrical charges of opposite sign, which could be eithr delocalized or non-delocalized, on adjacent or non-adjacent atoms.

Zygomorphic When the corolla or calyx could be divisible into equal halves in one plane only bilaterally symmetrical, with only one plane of symmetry.

Zygomycetes A type of fungi with coenocytic mycelium and chitinous cell wall. Its sexual reproduction usually engages the formation of zygospores.

Zygospore It is a sexual resting spore with thick wall which are characteristic of the zygomycetous fungi.

Zygote The diploid cell produced from the fusion of a male and female gamete during fertilisation.

Zygotic meiosis The meiosis which take place during the maturation or germination of zygote.